A clinical guide to implants in dentistry

A clinical guide to implants in dentistry

Edited by

Richard M. Palmer

Professor of Implant Dentistry and Periodontololgy,
Guy's, Kings and St Thomas' Medical and Dental Schools,
London

Principal authors

Peter D. Floyd
Leslie C. Howe
Paul J. Palmer

2000

Published by the British Dental Association
64 Wimpole Street, London, W1M 8AL

ISBN 0 904588 67 X

Printed and bound by Dennis Barber Graphics and Print,
Lowestoft, Suffolk

Foreword

The prime aim of this book is to present an overview of the application of osseointegrated implants in dental practice. It is not based upon a single implant system, but upon our experiences of a few well known and tested systems which have all produced highly successful and predictable results. It is not intended to be a step-by-step instruction manual of 'how to do it', but to give the clinician a wide appreciation of treatment planning, the various stages of treatment and how implant dentistry relates to and compares with other treatment options. There is a trend to present implant dentistry as a simple, straightforward procedure requiring minimal training. We trust that this book also demonstrates some of the complexities and pitfalls of this treatment modality, and the need for comprehensive education and training in this demanding field of dentistry.

We should like to thank the following people for their help: Vincent Barrett for his valuable contributions to Chapters 4, 7 and 9; David Radford (Department of Prosthetic Dentistry, GKT Dental School) for providing the electron microscopic images in Chapter 1; J Cawood , R Howell and Munksgaard International Publishers for permission to reproduce Figure 1c in Chapter 5; the highly skilled dental technicians who played an essential part in the treatment of our patients, and whose ideas have contributed to the development of this discipline; our postgraduate students for valuable academic and clinical interaction; Stephen Hancocks for his help with coordinating this project and to Peter Fyne for his efficient and expert planning and layout skills.

Richard M. Palmer
Peter D. Floyd
Leslie C. Howe
Paul J. Palmer
London, January 2000

Contents

Introduction to dental implants

Richard Palmer

Implants have been used to support dental prostheses for many decades, but they have not always enjoyed a favourable reputation. This situation has changed dramatically with the development of endosscous osscointegrated dental implants. They are the nearest equivalent replacement to the natural tooth, and are therefore a useful addition in the management of patients who have missing teeth because of disease, trauma or developmental anomalies. There are a number of dental implant systems which offer predictable long-term results backed by good scientific research and clinical trials. In the first place it may be helpful to clarify some of the commonly used terms in implant dentistry (Table 1).

Success criteria

It is important to establish success criteria for implant systems, and for implants to be tested in well controlled clinical trials. The minimum success criteria proposed by Albrektsson *et al.* (*IJOMI* 1986; **1**: 11) is set out in Table 2.

The most obvious sign of implant failure is mobility. However, some of the criteria in Table 2 apply to the overall requirements of an implant system, but are not as useful when judging the success of individual implants. This is well illustrated by considering the radiographic criteria. Bone remodelling occurs in the first year of function in response to occlusal forces and establishment of the normal dimensions of the peri-implant soft tissues (See Part 2). The 'ideal' bone level is usually judged against a specific landmark on the implant (such as the implant/abutment junction) and it may differ therefore between implant systems (fig. 6). Subsequently the bone levels are usually more or less stable, and small changes such as 0.2 mm per annum are impossible to measure with conventional radiographs. These specified changes therefore do not apply to individual implants but to mean (average) changes measured across a large number of implants. For example, a detectable change of 1mm or more may occur at very few implants in contrast to the majority which remain unchanged or in a steady state. It is also difficult to stipulate what level of change in an individual implant over a given period of time would constitute failure. A rapid change in bone level may be followed by a long period of stability. On the other hand, progressive or continuous bone loss is a worrying sign of impending failure. An implant with marked loss of bone may therefore be judged as 'surviving' rather than 'successful'.

Implants placed in the mandible (particularly anterior to the mental foramina) enjoy a higher success rate than the maxilla (approximately 95% success for implants in the

This first part of a new series outlines the salient aspects of osseointegration, implant design and other factors which contribute to successful treatment.

In this part, we will discuss:
- Success criteria
- Basic guide to osseointegration:
  - ➤ Biocompatibility and implant design
  - ➤ Bone factors
  - ➤ Loading conditions
  - ➤ Prosthetic considerations

Table 1	Basic terminology in implant dentistry
Osseointegration	A direct structural and functional connection between ordered, living bone and the surface of a load-carrying implant (Albrektsson *et al.* Acta Orthopaedica Scand 1981; **52**:155 (fig. 1).
Endosseous dental implant	A device inserted into the jaw bone (endosseous) to support a dental prosthesis. It is the 'tooth root' analogue and is often referred to as a 'fixture' (fig. 2).
Implant abutment	The component which attaches to the dental implant and supports the prosthesis. A transmucosal abutment (TMA) is one which passes through the mucosa overlying the implant. A temporary or healing abutment may be used during the healing of the peri-implant soft tissue before the definitive abutment is chosen (fig. 3).
Abutment screw	A screw used to connect an abutment to the implant.
Single stage implant surgery	Surgical placement of a dental implant which is left exposed to the oral cavity following insertion. This is the protocol used in non-submerged implant systems (fig. 4).
Two stage implant surgery	Initial surgical placement of a dental implant which is buried beneath the mucosa and then subsequently exposed with a second surgical procedure some months later. This is used in submerged implant systems (fig. 5).

dental implants

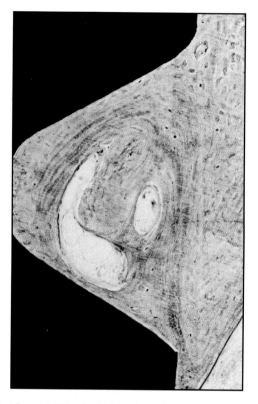

Figure 1. Histological section of an implant with bone growing in intimate contact with the surface. The dense bone which contains a small medullary space fills the area between two thread profiles which are 0.6 mm apart.

Implant design parameters
• Implant length
• Implant diameter
• Implant shape
• Surface characteristics

mandible compared with 85 to 90% for the maxilla with systems such as Branemark, 5 years after loading). An example of the lowest recorded success rates are for short implants (7 mm) used in the maxilla to support overdentures, especially when the implants are not joined together. A few studies have now shown that the overall mean failure rate in smokers is about twice that in non-smokers. Smokers should be warned of this association and encouraged to quit the habit. It should also be noted that reported mean failure rates are not evenly distributed throughout the patient population. Rather, implant failures are more likely to cluster in certain individuals.

Basic guide to osseointegration

Figure 1 shows an histological section of a titanium screw threaded implant which has been in function in bone for 1 year. There is very close apposition of bone over most of the implant surface. It has been proposed that the biological process leading to and maintaining osseointegration, is dependent upon a number of factors which include:

Biocompatibility and implant design

Implants made of commercially pure titanium have established a benchmark in osseointegration, against which few other materials compare. Related materials such as niobium are able to produce a high degree of osseointegration

Prosthetic considerations
• The type of prosthetic reconstruction
• The occlusal scheme
• The number, distribution, orientation, and design of implants
• The design and properties of implant connectors
• Dimensions and location of cantilever extensions
• Patient parafunctional activities

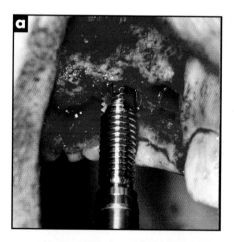

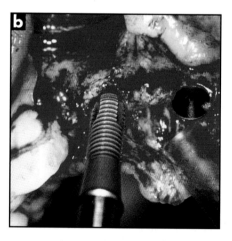

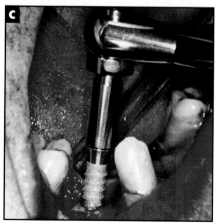

Figure 2. Three different designs of endosseous implants being inserted into prepared sites within the jaw bone. Scanning electron micrographs of the implants are shown in Figures 7 to 9. Figure 2a is a machined threaded implant of the Branemark design (Nobel Biocare). Figure 2b is an Astra ST implant which has a microthreaded coronal portion, a macro-threaded apical portion and the surface has been blasted with titanium oxide. Figure 2c is an ITI Straumann implant which has a smooth transmucosal collar, a macro-threaded body and a plasma sprayed surface.

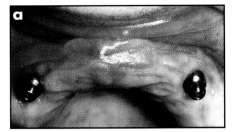
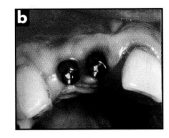
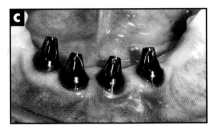
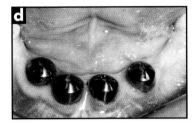

Figure 3. Various forms of implant abutment are illustrated. Figure 3a shows ball abutments which are used to support overdentures. Figure 3b shows abutments which are used to support individual crowns in 'single tooth restorations'. The crowns are cemented on the parallel sided hexagon. Figure 3c shows four conical shaped abutments which are used to support a bridge superstructure. In this the bridge would be screwed to the abutments rather than being cemented. Figure 3d shows some simple cylindrical healing abutments which are used during the healing phase of the mucosa before definitive abutments are selected.

and in addition, successful clinical results are reported for some titanium alloys and hydroxyapatite coated implants. More recently resorbable coatings have been developed which aim to improve the initial rate of bone healing against the implant surface and then resorb within a short time frame to allow establishment of a bone to metal contact.

The implant design has a great influence on initial stability and subsequent function. The main design parameters are:

- *Implant length* – implants are generally available in lengths from about 6 mm to as much as 20 mm. The most common lengths employed are between 8 and 15 mm which correspond quite closely to normal root lengths.
- *Implant diameter* — most implants are approximately 4 mm in diameter. At least 3.25 mm in diameter is required to ensure adequate implant strength. Implant diameter may be more important than implant length in the distribution of loads to the surrounding bone. Implant diameters up to 6 mm are available, which are considerably stronger, but they are not so widely used because sufficient bone width is not so commonly encountered.
- *Implant shape* — hollow-cylinders, solid-cylinders, hollow screws or solid screws are commonly employed shapes which are designed to maximise the potential area for

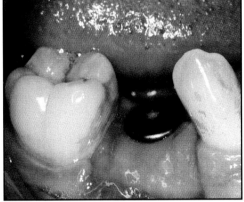

Figure 4. An implant of the ITI Straumann type has been inserted and left protruding through the mucosa in a one stage surgical procedure. A wide screw has been placed on the top to protect the inner aspect of the implant until a definitive abutment is connected.

osseointegration and provide good initial stability (figs 7a–9a). Even minor alterations in the size and pitch of threads can enhance the latter property. Screw shaped implants also offer good load distribution characteristics in function.

- *Surface characteristics* — the degree of surface roughness varies greatly between different systems. Surfaces which are machined, grit-blasted, etched, plasma sprayed and coated are available. Figures 7b to 9b show the characteristics of these surfaces viewed with the scanning electron microscope, showing considerable increases in potential surface area. The optimum surface morphology has yet to be defined, and some may perform better in certain circumstances. By

Table 2	Suggested minimum success criteria for dental implants*

1. An individual, unattached implant is immobile when tested clinically.
2. Radiographic examination does not reveal any peri-implant radiolucency.
3. After the first year in function, radiographic vertical bone loss is less than 0.2 mm per annum.
4. The individual implant performance is characterised by an absence of signs and symptoms such as pain, infections, neuropathies, paraesthesia, or violation of the inferior dental canal.
5. As a minimum, the implant should fulfil the above criteria with a success rate of 85% at the end of a 5 year observation period and 80% at the end of a 10 year period.

*after Albrektsson *et al.* IJOMI 1986; **1**:11

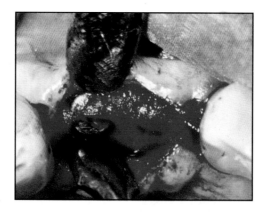

Figure 5. Exposure of two implants which have been buried beneath the mucosa for a period of 6 months. Bone has grown over the top of them and this needs to be removed before a healing abutment is connected.

increasing surface roughness there is the potential to increase the surface contact with bone but this may be at the expense of more ionic exchange and surface corrosion. Bacterial contamination of the implant surface will also be affected by the surface roughness if it becomes exposed within the mouth.

Bone factors

The stability of the implant at the time of placement is very important and is dependent upon bone quantity and quality as well as implant design. The edentulous ridge can be classified in terms of shape and bone quality (fig. 10). Following loss of a tooth the alveolar bone resorbs in width and height. In extreme cases bone resorption proceeds to a level which is beyond the normal extent of the alveolar process and well within the basal bone of the jaws. Radiographic determination of bone quantity and quality is considered in Part 5 and procedures which can be used to augment bone in Part 8. The most favourable quality of jaw bone for implant treatment is that which has a

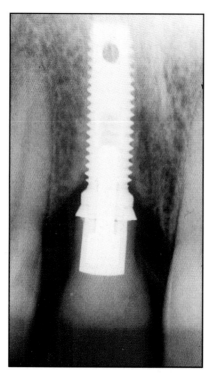

Figure 6. A periapical radiograph of a single tooth implant. The bone contacts the implant up to the most coronal thread. An abutment screw which is more radio-opaque can be seen connecting the abutment to the implant. The crown is all porcelain and is cemented to the abutment. In this system (Branemark) the landmark for measuring the bone level from is the junction between implant and abutment.

well formed cortex and densely trabeculated medullary spaces with a good blood supply. Bone which is predominantly cortical may offer good initial stability at implant placement but is more easily damaged by overheating during the drilling process, especially with sites more than 10 mm in depth. At the other extreme, bone with a thin or absent cortical layer and sparse trabeculation offers very poor initial implant stability and fewer cells with a good osteogenic potential to promote osseointegration. Success is highly dependent upon a surgical technique which avoids heating the bone. Slow drilling speeds, the use of successive incrementally larger sharp drills and copious saline irrigation aim to keep the temperature below that at which bone tissue damage occurs (around 47°C for 1 minute). Further refinements include cooling the irrigant and using internally irrigated drills. Methods by which these factors are controlled are considered in more detail in Part 6 (Basic Implant Surgery). Factors which compromise bone quality are infection, irradiation and heavy smoking. The effects of the latter two are a result of a diminution of the vascular supply to the bone which compromises the healing response, a feature which has been well described in the healing of fractures.

Loading conditions

Following installation of an implant it is important that it is not loaded during the early healing phase. Movement of the implant within the bone at this stage results in fibrous tissue encapsulation rather than osseointegration. This has been compared to the healing of a fracture where stabilisation of the bone fragments is very important to prevent non-union. In partially dentate subjects it is desirable to provide temporary/provisional prostheses which are tooth supported to avoid early implant loading. However, in patients who wear mucosally supported dentures it is generally recommended that they should not be worn over the implant area for 1 to 2 weeks. This also helps to prevent breakdown of the soft tissue wound. Systems such as Branemark have advised leaving implants unloaded beneath the mucosa for around 6 months in the maxilla and 3 months in the mandible, mainly because of differences in bone quality. However, these are largely empirical guidelines, and bone quality and implant stability will vary greatly between individuals, jaws and sites within jaws. Currently there is no accurate measure which precisely determines the optimum period of healing before loading can commence. Bone quality can be assessed by measuring the cutting torque during preparation of the implant site. The stability of an implant and increasing bone-to-implant contact has been quantified using resonance frequency analysis. This newly developed non-invasive research tool measures the stiffness of the implant at the bone interface. In some circumstances it has been shown that immediate loading is compatible with subsequent successful osseointegration, providing the bone quality is good and the functional forces can be adequately controlled. The latter may involve placing an adequate number of implants and connecting them together as soon as possible with a rigid framework. However, these latter protocols should be considered experimental at the present time, and there is much data to support the more cautious approach advocated by Branemark in ensuring a high level of predictable implant success. Some systems employ a single stage approach in which the implant is installed so that it protrudes through the overlying mucosa (ie non-submerged), although avoidance of early loading is equally critical. Following the recommended healing period (around 3 months) abutments are connected to the implant to allow construction of the prosthesis. This protocol therefore avoids further surgery to uncover the implants. The loading of the implant supported prosthesis is a further important consideration which will be dealt with in the following section.

Prosthetic considerations

Carefully planned functional occlusal loading will result in maintenance of osseointegration and possibly increased bone to implant contact. In contrast, excessive loading may lead to bone loss and/or component failure. Clinical loading conditions are largely dependent upon:

The type of prosthetic reconstruction

This can vary from a single tooth replacement in the partially dentate case to a full arch reconstruction in the edentulous individual. Implants which support overdentures may present particular problems with control of loading as they may be largely mucosal supported, entirely implant supported or a combination of the two.

The occlusal scheme

The lack of mobility in implant supported fixed prostheses requires provision of shallow cuspal inclines and careful distribution of loads in lateral excursions. With single tooth implant restorations it is important to develop initial tooth contacts on the natural dentition and to avoid guidance in lateral excursions on the implant restoration. Loading will also depend upon the opposing dentition which could be natural teeth, another implant supported prosthesis or a conventional removeable prosthesis. Surprisingly high forces can be generated through removable prostheses.

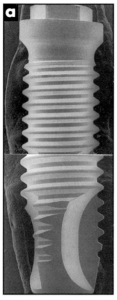
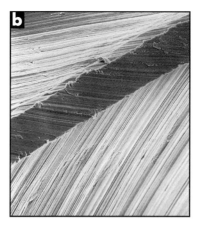

Figure 7. This shows a scanning electron micrograph of a Branemark/Nobel Biocare implant. Figure 7a shows the basic thread design and figure 7b a higher power view of the machined surface.

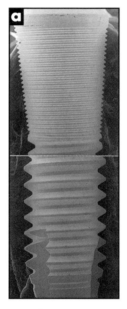
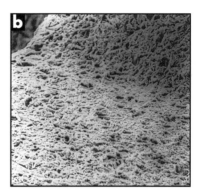

Figure 8 shows a scanning electron micrograph of an Astra ST implant. The conical neck has a microthread and the apical part a coarser self tapping thread (fig. 8a). Figure 8b shows a higher power view of the blasted (Tio-blast) surface at the same magnification as figure 7b.

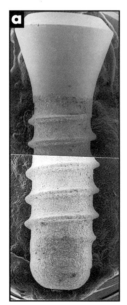
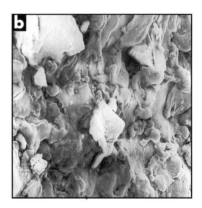

Figure 9 shows a scanning electron micrograph of an ITI Straumann solid screw implant. The polished transmucosal neck is clearly demarcated from the plasma sprayed body (fig. 9a). The thread has a coarser pitch than the implants shown in figures 7 and 8. Figure 9b shows the plasma sprayed surface at the same magnification as figure 7b and 8b. The increase in surface area is considerable.

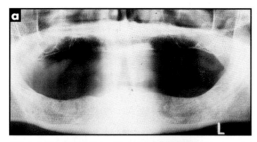

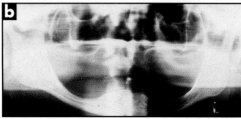

Figure 10 shows examples of dental panoramic tomograms of edentulous jaws. Both show extensive resorption of the maxillary ridge. There is far less resorption of the mandible in figure 10a than figure 10b. In the latter case there is reasonable bone volume in the anterior mandible but resorption close to the level of the inferior dental canal in the posterior part.

The number, distribution, orientation, and design of implants

The distribution of load to the supporting bone can be spread by increasing the number and dimensions (diameter, surface topography, length) of the implants. The spacing and 3-dimensional arrangement of the individual implants will also be very important. The so-called 'tripod' arrangement of three implants is recommended in situations of high load, such as replacement of molar teeth in the partially dentate individual.

The design and properties of implant connectors

Multiple implants are joined by a cast or milled framework. A rigid connector provides good splinting and distribution of loads between implants. It is equally important that the connector has a passive fit on the implant abutments so that loads are not set up within the prosthetic construction.

Dimensions and location of cantilever extensions. Some implant reconstructions are designed with cantilever extensions to provide function (and appearance) in areas where provision of additional implants is difficult. This may be caused by practical or financial considerations. Cantilever extensions have the potential to create high loads, particularly on the implant adjacent to the cantilever. The extent of the leverage of any cantilever should be considered in relation to the anteroposterior distance between implants supporting the reconstruction. The cantilever extension should not exceed this length and the cross sectional design should be adequate to prevent flexing.

Patient parafunctional activities

Great caution should be exercised in treating patients with known parafunctional activities. Excessive loads may lead to loss of marginal bone or component fracture.

These factors will be considered in more detail in Parts 4 and 7.

Conclusion

There are a great many factors to take into account to ensure predictable successful implant treatment. There is no substitute for meticulous attention to detail in all of these areas. Failure to do so will result in higher failure rates and unnecessary complications.

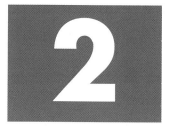

2 Teeth and implants

Richard Palmer

Clinicians who use dental implants in the treatment of their patients require an understanding of the nature of osseointegration and the important fundamental differences between dental implants and natural teeth. The main comparisons are summarised in Table 1 and illustrated in figure 1 which shows a single tooth implant and the adjacent natural teeth. The tooth originally formed within the jaws and erupted through the overlying mucosa in a complex series of biological events that are by no means fully understood. The implant on the other hand was surgically placed within the jaw bone, and is one of the few prosthetic devices that has been shown to successfully and permanently breach the surface epithelium with minimal or no complications.

Gingiva versus periimplant soft tissues

In healthy teeth the gingival margin is located on enamel. The gingival margin is scalloped and forms a shallow sulcus at the tooth surface. The gingiva rises between the teeth to form the interdental papillae, which are complex structures. Between the anterior teeth the papillae are pyramidal structures with the attachment of the gingivae following the contour of the cement enamel junction (fig. 2). In the molar regions, the buccal and lingual papillae at natural tooth embrasures are separated by the 'col', an area of gingivae which forms a slight dip beneath the contact point. A complex array of

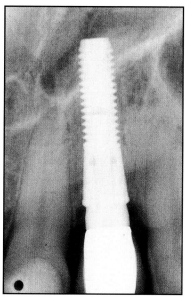

Fig. 1b Radiograph of the single tooth implant and adjacent teeth. The bone contacts the implant surface with no intervening radiolucent space which would be observed if there were fibrous tissue encapsulation. The bone margin is coincident with the implant/abutment junction. The adjacent teeth have a normal periodontal ligament space

gingival connective tissue fibres form well defined bundle groups:

· Interdental fibres
· Dento-gingival fibres
· Circular fibres
· Alveolar crest fibres.

Many of these fibres are inserted into the root cementum between the alveolar crest and cement enamel junction, and are therefore dependent upon the presence of natural teeth.

In the case of an implant, a transmucosal element (an abutment, neck of the implant or the restoration) protrudes through the overlying mucosa which heals and adapts around it without a cementum attachment. The collagen fibres within the periimplant mucosa run parallel to the abutment with no insertion into the abutment surface. There have been descriptions of more ordered fibre arrangements in relation to transmucosal implant surfaces which have a rougher surface (such as plasma spraying). In this situation some fibres appear to run at right angles to the implant surface, but there is no good evidence of an attachment mechanism. However a rough abutment surface does have potential negative properties,

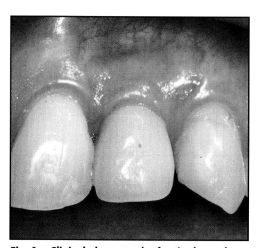

Fig. 1a. Clinical photograph of a single tooth implant replacing the upper left lateral incisor. The porcelain fused to metal crown appears to emerge from the gingiva with interdental tissue which appears very similar to normal papillae

An osseointegrated implant restoration may closely resemble a natural tooth. However, the absence of a periodontal ligament and connective tissue attachment via cementum, results in fundamental differences in the adaptation of the implant to occlusal forces, and the structure of the gingival cuff.

In this part, we will discuss:
● Gingiva versus periimplant soft tissues
● Periodontal ligament versus osseointegration
● Periodontitis and peri-implantitis

Table 1	Healthy teeth versus healthy implants	
	Healthy teeth	**Healthy implants**
Gingival sulcus depth	Shallow in health	Dependent upon abutment length and restoration margin
Junctional epithelium	On enamel	On titanium
Gingival fibres	Complex array inserted into cementum above crestal bone	No organised collagen fibre attachment – parallel fibres
Crest of bone	1 to 2 mm apical to CEJ	According to implant design eg at or about first thread in threaded implants or at the level of change in surface morphology
Connective tissue attachment	Well organised collagen fibre bundles inserted as Sharpey's fibres into alveolar bone and cementum	Bone growing into close contact with implant surface: oxide layer/ bone proteoglycan and collagen
Physical characteristics	Physiologic mobility caused by viscoelastic properties of the ligament	Rigid connection to bone - as if ankylosed
Adaptive characteristics	Width of ligament can alter to allow more mobility with increased occlusal forces	No adaptive capacity to allow mobility. Orthodontic movement impossible
Proprioception	Highly sensitive receptors present within the periodontal ligament	No ligament receptors

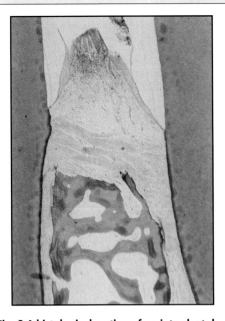

Fig. 2 A histological section of an interdental space between two teeth. The enamel has been removed by the demineralisation process. The junctional epithelium outlines the enamel space and terminates at the level of the root cementum. The interdental bone septum is situated just below the cement enamel junction (in health 1–2 mm) and there is a well developed transeptal fibre arrangement. There is a small inflammatory infiltrate in the gingival connective tissue at the top of the papilla

such as increased corrosion potential and microbial contamination if it becomes exposed within the oral cavity.

The papillae which form around a single tooth implant may be supported by collagen fibres attached to the adjacent natural teeth. However, in cases where there are adjacent implants rather than teeth, the formation of soft tissue papillae is less predictable and their form is dependent upon the presence of an adequate thickness of soft tissue, bone height, implant spacing and careful contouring of the crown profiles to encourage the appearance and maintenance of a papillary form (fig. 3). The soft tissue between multiple posterior unit implants is more likely to have a flat contour but again may be influenced by soft tissue thickness and crown morphology.

Junctional epithelium

In healthy teeth the junctional epithelium (fig. 4) is attached to enamel by hemidesmosomal contacts and a basal lamina-like structure formed by the epithelial cells. The biological attachment mechanism is now thought to be mediated through particular adhesins or integrins, which are fundamental in cell to cell adhesion as well as cell to matrix adhesion. It is well established that a junctional epithelium will also form on root surface cementum, dentine and various dental materials including implant components (fig. 5). A normal junctional epithelium can be regenerated from adjacent oral mucosa/gingiva following excision, and the new junctional epithelium is indistinguishable from that which previously existed. It is thought that the properties of the junctional epithelium are dictated by the influence of the underlying connective tissue, the presence of an inflammatory infiltrate and the presence of a tooth/implant surface to which it adheres (rather than the inherent properties of the epithelial cells). The junctional epithelium has a particularly high turnover and is permeable to both the ingress of substances and to components of the immune and inflammatory system. It is therefore well equipped to deal with the problems of a breach in the epithelial integrity caused by an emerging tooth or implant. The junctional epithelium may be found on the implant itself or on the abutment. This will be because of differences in the designs of implants, the biological requirements of the attachment of the soft tissue cuff and the level of the junction between abutment and implants.

Biological width

In teeth, the concept of the biological width is well established, in that a zone of attached connective tissue separates the underlying alveolar bone from the apical termination of the junctional epithelium (fig. 6a). The connective tissue zone is about 2 mm wide and the length of the junctional epithelium about 1.5 mm. Figures 6b and c show two different designs of implants and the corresponding biological width. In the first case the implant design is typical of a submerged (two stage) system such as the Branemark. After 1 year of function the bone margin is usually located at the first thread. The junctional epithelium (1.5 mm to 2 mm apicocoronal width) is located on the abutment, and a zone of non-arranged connective tissue of about 1mm to 2 mm in width intervenes. The join between abutment and implant head is located within this zone. In contrast the non-submerged (single stage) implant (typical of the ITI Straumann type) is placed so that its roughened surface is placed within bone, but the smooth neck which is an integral part of the implant performs the function of the transmucosal element. The junctional epithelium is therefore routinely located on the implant, and the implant/abutment join is located coronal to this level. It has been postulated that the join within the submerged (two stage) system may influence the level of soft tissue attachment and biological width. This may be caused by micromovement between the two components or by allowing microbial penetration of the microgap between

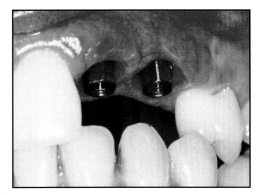

Figure 3a. Two hexagonal abutments used to support single implant crowns emerging through a cuff of gingiva. The space around them has been created by a larger healing abutment which has been replaced by the hexagonal abutment. The gingival tissue between the abutments has a form which resembles a normal papilla but is flatter and is not supported by a normal gingival fibre arrangement

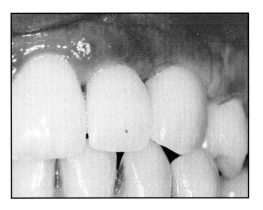

Fig. 3b The porcelain fused to metal crowns have been cemented onto the abutments. The emergence of the crowns from the soft tissue produces a natural looking appearance

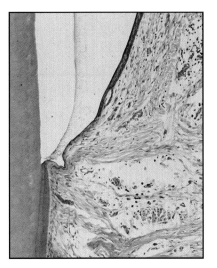

Fig. 4. A histological section of junctional epithelium at a natural tooth. It terminates at the cement enamel junction and was attached to the enamel by hemidesmosomes and a basal lamina-like structure. Collagen fibres are inserted into the cementum and radiate into the gingival connective tissue

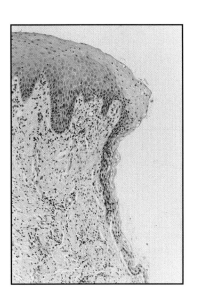

Fig. 5 A histological section of the soft tissue cuff excised from around an implant. A non-keratinised sulcular and junctional epithelium is present and is very similar to that which exists around teeth. The collagen fibre bundles are not so well organised as there is no attachment to the abutment/implant surface

dental implants

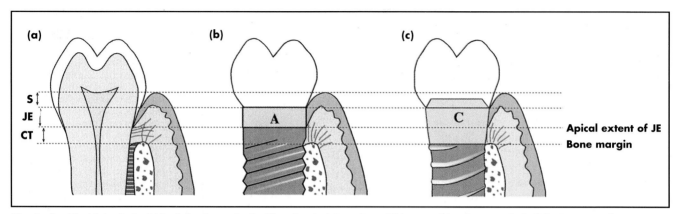

Fig. 6 a,b,c The biological width of the dentogingival junction in (a) teeth and (b) around implants typical of the Branemark system, and (c) the non-submerged ITI implant system. S= sulcus which is approximately 0.5 to 1 mm deep; JE = junctional epithelium which is about 1.5 to 2 mm in apicocoronal width; CT = Connective tissue zone (1 to 2 mm in width) in which the fibres are attached to root cementum in teeth but run parallel to the implant surface; A = abutment — The abutment to implant junction is situated beneath the soft tissue in the Branemark system; C = smooth transmucosal collar of the IT system

Periodontal ligament versus osseointegration
- Periodontal ligament
- Osseointegration

implant and abutment. At present the theoretical differences between the two types do not reveal any major differences at the histological level or in their clinical performance.

Probing depth examination

Periodontal probing of natural teeth is an important part of any dental examination. It is well established that the probe penetrates the junctional epithelium to some degree in health, and that this penetration increases in the presence of inflammation. Under these latter circumstances the probe is stopped by the most coronal intact gingival connective tissue fibres, about 2 mm from the bone. The situation around the dental implant is different and the sulcus depth is very much dependent upon the thickness of the soft tissue cuff. Probing depths around implants are generally deeper than around teeth, but penetration of the soft tissue at the base of the sulcus occurs to a similar degree with the probe tip finishing short of the bone margin by about 2 mm. The information gained from probing around implants is of questionable value and many clinicians do not

recommend probing, preferring to rely on radiographic assessment of bone levels. In addition, digital pressure on the external surface of the periimplant soft tissue may elicit signs of inflammation such as bleeding or suppuration.

Periodontal ligament versus osseointegration

Periodontal ligament

The periodontal ligament is a complex structure, about 0.1 to 0.2 mm in width, providing support to the teeth in a viscoelastic manner (fig. 7). The ligament comprises collagen fibres which are embedded as Sharpey's fibres in the root cementum and the alveolar bone, together with the blood supply and connective tissue ground substance which provide the other key elements to the supporting mechanism. The periodontal ligament has a sensitive proprioceptive mechanism which can detect minute changes in forces applied to the teeth. Forces applied to the teeth are dissipated through compression and redistribution of the fluid elements as well as through the fibre system. Forces transmitted through the periodontal ligament can result in remodelling and tooth movement as seen in orthodontics or in the widening of the ligament and an increase in tooth mobility in response to excessive forces (eg occlusal trauma). The periodontal ligament is therefore capable of detecting and responding to a wide range of forces.

Osseointegration

The precise nature of osseointegration at a molecular level is not fully understood. At the light microscopical level there is a very close adaptation of the bone to the implant surface (fig. 8). At the higher magnifications possible with electron microscopy, there is a gap (about 100 NM in width) between the implant surface and bone. This is occupied by an intervening collagen rich zone adjacent to the bone and a more amor-

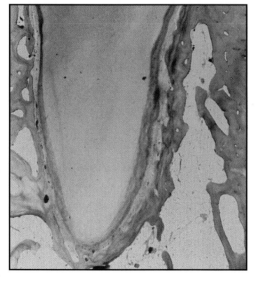

Fig. 7 A histological section of a tooth root, periodontal ligament and alveolar bone. The periodontal ligament is inserted into the cementum and the lamina dura as Sharpey's fibres. The viscoelastic properties of the ligament give the tooth a degree of mobility and the ligament is able to respond to increased forces by remodelling processes

phous zone adjacent to the implant surface. Bone proteoglycans may be important in the initial attachment of the tissues to the implant surface, which in the case of titanium implants consists of a titanium oxide layer, which has the properties of a ceramic. Osseointegration is not an absolute phenomenon and can be measured as the proportion of the total implant surface that is in contact with bone. Greater levels of bone contact occur in cortical bone than in cancellous bone, where marrow spaces are often adjacent to the implant surface. The degree of bone contact may increase with time and function. When an implant is first placed in the bone there should be a close fit to ensure stability. The space between implant and bone is initially filled with blood clot and serum/bone proteins. Although great care is taken to avoid damaging the bone, the initial response to the surgical trauma is resorption, which is then followed by bone deposition. There is a critical period in the healing process at around 2 weeks post implant insertion when bone resorption will result in a lower degree of implant stability than that achieved initially. Subsequent bone formation will result in an increase in the level of bone contact and stability. This has been demonstrated in unloaded implants in the early healing period and over longer time periods following loading of the implant. Thus osseointegration should be viewed as a dynamic process in which bone turnover occurs, but not as the same adaptive process that occurs within the ligament of natural teeth. Osseointegration is more akin to an ankylosis, where the absence of mobility and no intervening fibrous tissue capsule is the sign of successful integration. Under these circumstances there is no viscoelastic damping system although proprioceptive mechanisms may operate within bone and associated oral structures. Forces are distributed to the bone and may be concentrated in certain areas, particularly around the neck of the implant. Some designs, particularly those with threads, may dissipate the forces more effectively. Excessive forces applied to the implant may result in remodelling of the marginal bone ie apical movement of the bone margin with loss of osseointegration. The exact mechanism of how this occurs is not entirely clear but it has been suggested that microfractures may propogate within the adjacent bone. This type of bone loss caused by excessive loading may be slowly progressive to a point where there is catastrophic failure of the remaining osseointegration or fracture of the implant. Fortunately, either eventuality is rare. Excessive forces are usually detected prior to this stage through radiographic marginal bone loss or mechanical failure of the superstructure and/or abutments (See Part 10).

It has been shown however, that well controlled forces result in an increase in the degree of bone to implant contact and remodelling of

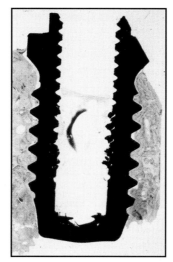 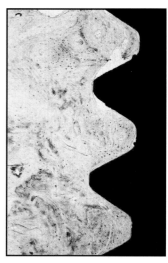

Fig. 8a A histological section through an osseointegrated screw shaped implant which has been in place for 6 months. Bone is in close apposition over a large proportion of the surface

Fig. 8b A higher power view of an area of figure 8a showing bone filling the thread profiles and contacting the implant surface without a visible gap (at this magnification), except for a small area of marrow space

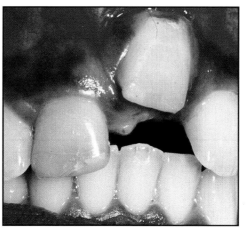

Fig. 9 An ankylosed tooth following trauma. Damage to the periodontal ligament has led to a boney ankylosis and resorption. The tooth has no detectable mobility and has not developed into a normal vertical position with the adjacent teeth. In this respect it is behaving like an osseointegrated implant. An osseointegrated implant should not be placed in a child until growth is complete

adjacent trabecular structures to dissipate the forces. Adaptation is therefore possible, though osseointegration does not permit movement of the implant in the way that a tooth may be orthodontically repositioned. Therefore the osseointegrated implant has proved itself to be a very effective anchorage system for difficult orthodontic cases, and may be used as an alternative anchorage system to head gear. The fact that the implant behaves as an ankylosed unit also restricts its use to individuals who have completed their jaw growth (fig. 9). Placement of an osseointegrated implant in a child will result in relative submergence with growth of the surrounding alveolar process during normal development. It is therefore advisable to delay implant placement until after growth is complete.

Periodontitis and peri-implantitis
It is quite possible that bacteria which are implicated in periodontitis, such as *Porphryromonas gingivalis*, are also the major pathogens in destructive inflammatory lesions around implants (peri-implantitis). There is

dental implants

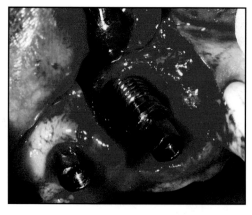

Fig. 10 An exposed implant following destruction of the most coronal bone by an inflammatory infiltrate. There was a plaque induced inflammation caused by retention of cement at the crown abutment junction which was situated subgingivally

therefore a possibility of colonisation or infection of the implant surfaces from pre-existing periodontopathic bacteria. The destruction of the supporting tissues of teeth and implants have many similarities but there are important differences caused by the nature of the supporting tissues (see earlier). This is particularly noticeable with the different patterns of tissue destruction observed. Peri-implantitis affects the entire circumference of the implant resulting in a 'gutter' of bone loss filled with inflammatory tissue extending to the bone surface (fig. 10). In contrast, periodontitis-affected teeth commonly have irregular loss of supporting tissues, often confined to proximal surfaces and resulting in complex infrabony defects. In addition, for the most part the periodontal tissues are capable of 'walling off' the inflammatory lesion from the alveolar bone and periodontal ligament with a zone of fibrous tissue. It would seem probable that destructive inflammatory lesions affecting both teeth and implants have stages in which the disease process is more rapid (burst phenomenon) followed by periods of relative quiescence. The incidence of peri-implantitis would appear to be low, but can result in rapid destruction of the marginal bone and is difficult to differentiate from bone loss because of excessive forces. This problem is dealt with in Part 10.

Conclusion

Modern osseointegrated implants are a useful alternative to natural teeth. There are fundamental differences between them, and an understanding of the attachment mechanisms of hard and soft tissues and their responses to the harsh environment of the oral cavity is essential to the dental surgeon who is involved in providing this form of treatment.

3 Assessment of the dentition and treatment options for the replacement of missing teeth

Richard Palmer,[1] and Leslie Howe,[2]

The restorative dentist has a wide range of options for replacement of teeth lost through dental disease, trauma or causes such as developmental anomalies.

The most common causes of tooth loss are dental caries (and its sequelae) and periodontal disease. Both diseases have an impact on the condition and prognosis of the remaining teeth which will therefore require very careful assessment to determine whether they require remedial treatment and furthermore whether they would provide suitable abutments for fixed or removable prostheses. It is essential that all caries, endodontic lesions and periodontal disease have been treated before embarking on definitive replacement of missing teeth by whatever method is finally chosen.

Initial examination and considerations

The minimal clinical examination should assess the restorative status of the teeth, a periodontal screening, mucous membranes, TMJs, jaw relationship and occlusion. Vitality testing should also be carried out where appropriate and a complete periodontal examination for all those whose screening indicates significant periodontitis (BPE score 4 in any sextant) (fig. 1).

The most convenient overall radiographic examination is the dental panoramic tomogram (fig. 2). This may need to be supplemented with intra-oral radiographs where the

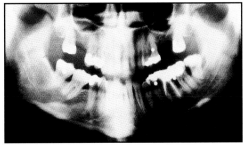

Fig. 2 The dental panoramic tomogram is a very useful screening tool. This individual has a heavily restored dentition and moderate to advanced periodontitis. The image in the mid-line is not quite so clear but it does indicate advanced bone loss on the incisor teeth

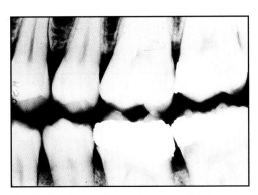

Fig. 3 Bitewing radiographs are useful for diagnosis of caries and early periodontal disease. Recurrent caries is visible on the mesial aspect of the lower second molar but the interdental bone crests are at a normal level

image quality does not permit proper assessment. Bitewing radiographs are adequate for dentitions minimally affected by caries or early periodontitis (fig. 3). Periapical radiographs using a paralleling technique should be considered advisable for all potential abutment teeth, heavily restored teeth, teeth with known or suspected endodontic problems and teeth with moderate to advanced periodontitis (fig. 4).

Following a full clinical and radiographic examination, it may be helpful to assign a prognosis to individual teeth , taking into account all factors: restorative, endodontic, periodontal. The prognosis may be simply categorised eg excellent/good, fair, questionable/poor, hopeless. In addition, the individual tooth prognosis may be affected by the type of planned restoration. For example, a tooth with a post crown

In most cases the patient and dentist have a number of choices for the replacement of missing teeth. The advantages and disadvantages of these options can be presented following careful clinical and radiographic examinations.

In this part, we will discuss:
- Initial examination and considerations
- Potential abutment teeth
- The edentulous area
- Advantages and disadvantages of treatment options
- Treatment choices

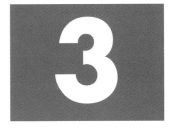

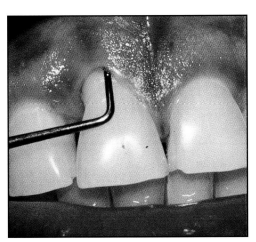

Fig. 1 Probing to assess the periodontal status of the patient. In this case a relatively healthy looking gingival margin has a probing depth of nearly 10 mm

[1]*Professor of Implant Dentistry and Periodontology, Guy's Kings and St Thomas' Medical and Dental School, London SE1 9RT* [2]*Consultant in Restorative Dentistry, Guy's and St Thomas' Hospital Trust, and Specialist in Restorative Dentistry and Prosthodontics, 21 Wimpole Street, London W1M 7AD*

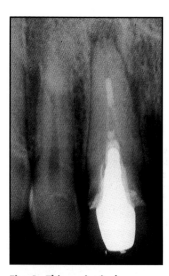

Fig. 4a This periapical radiograph shows an upper right central incisor with an inadequate root filling, an apical radiolucency and a very short post. This tooth would not be considered to be a suitable bridge abutment

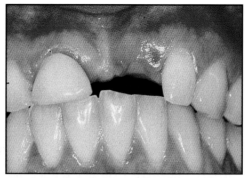

Fig. 4b The clinical status of the patient illustrated in figure 4a. The missing upper left central incisor space is large. The patient had a mid-line diastema prior to tooth loss

tion of the edentulous space and the occlusal relationships will have a great effect on the possible restorative solutions.

Potential abutment teeth

The size and shape of the natural crown and root form are important considerations.

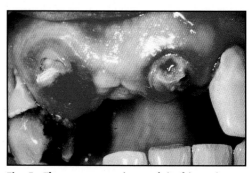

Fig. 5a The upper anterior teeth in this patient are very broken down. They were bridge abutments which have suffered from caries and fracture. Restoration of these teeth would be very difficult. If individual restorations were possible it is unlikely that they would be considered to be adequate bridge abutments

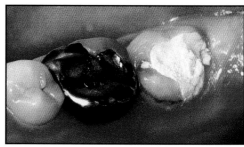

Fig. 5b The first and second molars are heavily restored. The second molar requires a replacement restoration but this extends subgingivally to a considerable extent. This retromolar area is difficult to perform periodontal surgery to expose restoration margins

may have a fair prognosis if it is to be kept as a free standing unit, but would be severely compromised if used to support a denture or fixed bridge. Features which adversely affect the prognosis are described in Table 1 and illustrated in figure 5.

The basic questions to be asked about individual teeth are:
1. Can the tooth be restored successfully?
2. Can the tooth be endodontically treated successfully?
3. Can the tooth be treated periodontally?
4. Following treatment will the tooth be a suitable abutment?
5. How important is the tooth strategically?
6. What impact will the loss of the tooth have on the overall plan?

The individual tooth assessment and prognosis then needs to be put into the context of the treatment requirements of the entire dentition. In addition to the above considerations, many subjects are seen with missing teeth due to trauma or developmental absence of teeth in whom the remaining dentition is very healthy. The potential abutment teeth, the size and loca-

Table 1	Important factors which adversely affect individual tooth prognosis
Restorations and caries	Extensions subgingivally or onto root surfaces
	Extension within the pulp chamber or root canal
	Minimal remaining coronal tooth substance
	Inadequate or overextended posts in root filled teeth
Endodontic factors	Periapical symptoms/signs
	Inability to control the coronal seal
	Inadequate previous RCT including broken instruments in root canal
	Sclerosed canals
	Fractures/splits
Periodontal factors	Probing depths over 6 mm
	Attachment loss over 6 mm
	Bone loss, more than 50%
	Poor root morphology — especially short roots
	Involvement of furcations — especially grade II/III
	Mobility — especially grade III
Occlusal factors	
	Signs of parafunction or severe attrition
	History of repeated tooth restoration/fractures

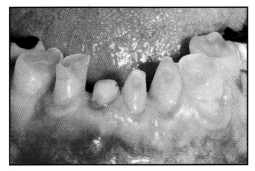

Fig. 5c These heavily worn teeth have been crown lengthened but restoration is still difficult. The lower right central incisor is non-vital and has a labial sinus. This tooth was considered to be untreatable

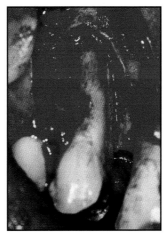

Fig. 5d This shows surgical exposure of a complex bone defect affecting the upper right first pre-molar. A deep periodontal pocket was detected on the mesial aspect in relation to the groove and the bifurcation of this tooth. Recurrent abscesses have destroyed most of the buccal and mesial bone. This tooth has a very poor prognosis

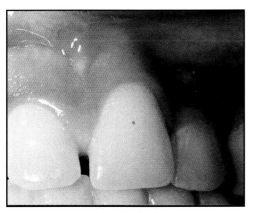

Fig. 6a This patient had orthodontic treatment to close space following loss of an upper central incisor. The upper right lateral incisor is now in the position of the central incisor. The gingival margins are at different levels

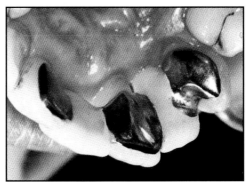

Fig. 7a A palatal view of a Maryland bridge replacing maxillary incisor teeth. The casting covers as much of the palatal enamel as possible to improve the retention, but care has to be taken to avoid interference with the incisal guidance

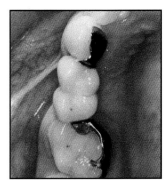

Fig. 7b A Maryland bridge used to replace the upper first and second pre-molars. Seat rests have been prepared to prevent apical displacement and the casting wraps around the palatal aspects of the abutment teeth

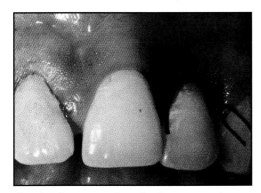

Fig. 6b Minor crown lengthening surgery has been performed on both upper lateral incisors to improve the aesthetics and allow restoration of the upper right lateral to match that of the upper left central incisor

Teeth with short and conical crown forms offer poor retention and support. Procedures such as periodontal surgical crown lengthening or adhesive restorations may overcome many of the difficulties (figs 6 and 7). Certain teeth, particularly canines, are very difficult to replace with routine restorations because of the lack of suitable adjacent abutments (fig. 8). Loss of the canine in a distal free end saddle situation leaves only the lateral incisor as a distal abutment for a removable prosthe-sis. This is a most unsatisfactory situation and often leads to progressive loss of the incisors (fig. 9).

Healthy unrestored teeth make the best abutments for fixed bridges but the damage that occurs to teeth following preparation must be considered. Conversely heavily restored teeth may be unsuitable abutments. Further tooth preparation may remove the only remaining

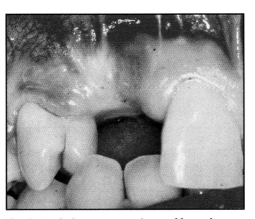

Fig. 8. A missing upper canine and lateral incisor. The lateral incisor was developmentally absent and a transplantation of the canine into the space failed. Restoration of this space is extremely difficult

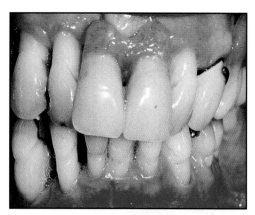

Fig. 9 A patient who has suffered from extensive periodontal disease. The missing upper teeth have been replaced with a removable partial denture. The lower right canine has a poor prognosis and this is the most distal tooth in the lower right quadrant. Loss of this tooth will present considerable difficulties with provision of a removable restoration, and the prognosis of the lower incisors will be affected

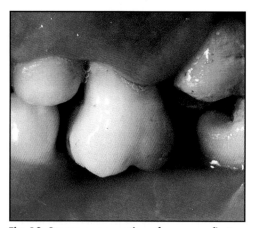

Fig. 10. Severe overeruption of an upper first molar into the opposing edentulous space

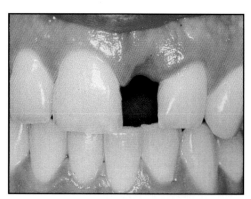

Fig. 11 Following loss of the upper left central incisor there has been considerable space closure and simple provision of a replacement tooth with normal dimensions is not possible

tooth substance and restorations retained by pins or posts are prone to failure.

The edentulous area

The requirements for restoring an edentulous area depend upon its location and size. Many subjects will accept or prefer non-replacement of missing molars. The concept of the shortened arch is well established and most patients will accept a dentition extending from first molar to first molar or from second premolar to second premolar. Patients with fewer teeth than this often have an aesthetic problem and functional disadvantage. The point at which replacement of missing posterior teeth in the free end saddle situation is carried out is very much dependent upon patient wishes. The alternative to an implant supported prosthesis is a removable prosthesis or a limited extension distal cantilever bridge. Replacement of molar teeth to prevent over-eruption of teeth in the opposing arch, which may compromise future restorative options, is important in some subjects (fig. 10).

Few patients will accept non-replacement of missing incisors/canines. The full range of prosthetic options can be considered and an explanation of their advantages and disadvantages given to the patient. There are, however, a few general considerations.

Single missing teeth

The size of the edentulous space of single missing units varies enormously. At one extreme there is barely enough space for the missing unit (fig. 11). Orthodontic realignment may need to be considered to either eliminate the space or provide enough to accommodate the missing unit (fig. 12). In other cases the single

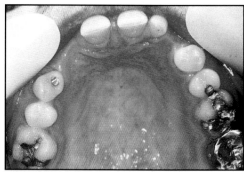

Fig. 12a This individual has a number of developmentally absent teeth, spacing between the incisors and rotation of the upper right premolar

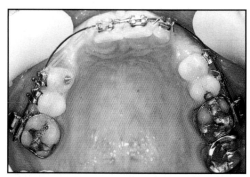

Fig. 12b Improvement of the spacing and rotations following orthodontic treatment

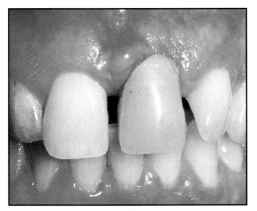

Fig. 13a Replacement of the upper left central incisor with a removable denture

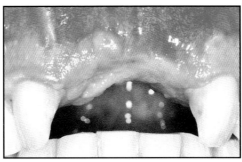

Fig. 14a An anterior edentulous space with loss of ridge height in the mid-line. Replacement of the missing tissue would be necessary to achieve a satisfactory aesthetic result. This may be achieved using surgical reconstruction or as part of the prosthesis

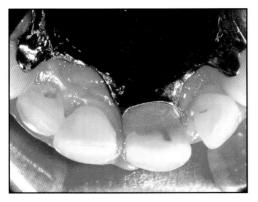

Fig. 13b Palatal view of the same individual showing extensive coverage of the palatal tissue by the chrome cobalt framework. Replacement of an incisor in a spaced dentition may be achieved using a removable denture, a spring cantilevered bridge or a single tooth implant

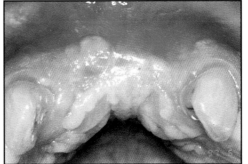

Fig. 14b The same ridge seen from the occlusal aspect showing a concavity on the patient's left side following loss of the buccal plate when the tooth was avulsed

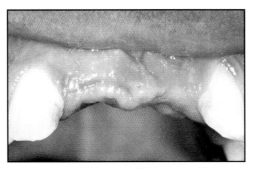

Fig. 15a Loss of the central incisors in this patient has led to minimal ridge resorption

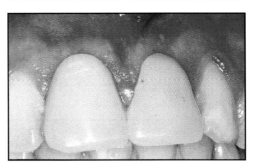

Fig. 15b The same patient with a provisional acrylic denture with ridge lapped teeth showing very good aesthetics

tooth space may be larger than the natural tooth. In spaced dentitions the prosthetic options for replacement of the single missing tooth are more limited (fig. 13).

Multiple missing teeth

In many cases patients will present with an existing prosthesis which gives information about the aesthetic requirements, including the number and size of teeth which can be accommodated. In other cases it will be necessary to carry out a diagnostic wax-up or provision of a temporary denture to establish this. The height and shape of the edentulous ridge is another important consideration. It should be remembered that following tooth loss, alveolar resorption may occur in both a horizontal and vertical plane (fig. 14). Factors which influence the degree of resorption include previous periodontal and endodontic infections, surgical trauma during extraction, postoperative infection, and the type and quality of the previous prosthesis. Loss of ridge height and width may necessitate prosthetic replacement of the missing soft and hard tissues to provide adequate aesthetics at the gingival margin and lip sup-port. In removable prostheses this can be achieved with a labial flange but if a fixed restoration is to be chosen, then some form of ridge augmentation may be necessary. The pro-

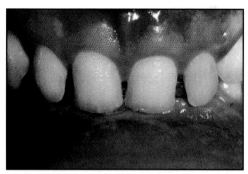

Fig. 16a A severe Class II division 2 incisor relationship with the upper teeth biting into the opposing ridge

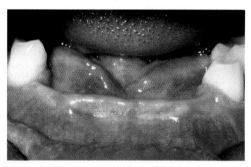

Fig. 16b The opposing ridge which has indentations from the upper incisors

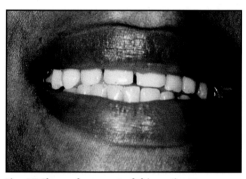

Fig. 17 The replacement of this patient's upper incisor teeth with a removable prosthesis produces an entirely satisfactory aesthetic result. The intra-oral views of this denture are shown in figure 22b

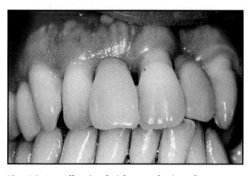

Fig. 18 An adhesive bridge replacing the upper right central and upper left lateral incisors in a patient who has undergone periodontal treatment. This restoration produces a very good aesthetic result, although some greying of the incisor tips of the abutment teeth is visible

vision of a diagnostic temporary denture may be advisable to determine whether a labial flange is needed (fig. 15).

Occlusal relationships

Examination of the occlusion should encompass basic jaw relationships and determination of the intercuspal position. The patient's mandible should be manipulated into its most retruded position and the presence of any contacts in this retruded arc should be sought. Movement of the mandible laterally and anteriorly should demonstrate the existing occlusal relationships and presence of any significant interferences. For individuals with edentulous spans greater than one unit it is advisable to take accurate study casts and mount these in a semi-adjustable articulator using a facebow. This will allow a clear assessment of the occlusal scheme and implications of the treatment alternatives to be more accurately assessed.

Some cases, such as Class 2 division 2 incisor relationships, can pose particularly difficult problems with any type of prosthesis due to space and angulation limitation (Figure 16). Tilted and overerupted teeth may need to be corrected before a satisfactory restoration can be provided. Restoration of individuals with parafunctional activities or severe occlusal wear demand special care.

Advantages and disadvantages of treatment options

Removeable prostheses

These are a commonly prescribed treatment option and may be used as a long term restoration or provisional restoration prior to a fixed prosthesis (fig. 17).

Advantages
- Replace multiple teeth in multiple sites
- Support obtained from mucosa and/or teeth
- Generally do not require extensive preparation of abutment teeth
- May be designed to accommodate future tooth loss
- Can be used to replace missing soft tissue
- Can provide good lip support by incorporating labial flanges
- Aesthetics may be very good
- The least expensive of restorations

Disadvantages
- Removeable prostheses may not be liked by patient and may reduce self-confidence
- Connectors cover soft tissue such as the palate and gingiva
- In subjects with less than ideal oral hygiene they may compromise the health of the periodontal tissues and promote caries around abutment teeth

- Retentive elements such as clasps may spoil aesthetics
- Moderate maintenance requirements and durability.

Fixed prostheses
Fixed prostheses fall into two main categories
1. Resin bonded bridgework (fig. 18)
2. Conventional partial or full coverage bridge-work (fig. 19)

Resin bonded bridgework

Advantages
- Minimal or no preparation required
- Fixed restoration
- Good aesthetics if ideal spacing exists and abutment teeth are satisfactory
- Less expensive than conventional bridges
- Consequences of failure are relatively small - caries is readily diagnosed in most instances. Cantilever designs for single tooth replacements minimise potential problems

Disadvantages
- Lack of predictability: decementation leading to loss of retention or caries under one of the retainers — average life span 5 to 7 years.
- Dependent upon meticulous technique and available enamel surface area for bonding
- Change in colour/translucency of abutment teeth due to presence of retainer
- May interfere with occlusion, particularly incisal guidance
- Patients may feel sense of insecurity with restoration, especially if their bridge has debonded previously

Conventional partial or full coverage bridgework

Advantages
- Fixed
- Good appearance, including that of abutment teeth if they need to be improved/harmonised
- Medium term predictability is good for short span bridges
- Good control of occlusion possible
- Minimally compromise oral hygiene

Disadvantages
- Involve considerable tooth preparation which sometimes result in pulpal sequelae
- Failure due to decementation and caries of abutment teeth may lead to further tooth loss
- Moderately expensive
- Highly operator dependent requiring exacting techniques both clinically and technically
- Requires lengthy clinical time and temporary restorations
- Irreversible

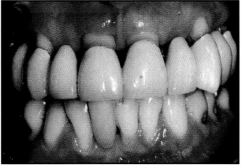
Fig. 19 A full arch fixed bridge in a patient who had lost many of her upper teeth through periodontitis. This design of bridge is an effective splint for the remaining teeth which have very much reduced periodontal support. The lower right central incisor has been replaced with an adhesive bridge

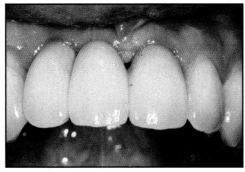
Fig. 20a The anterior view of an implant retained bridge replacing the upper right lateral incisor and both central incisors

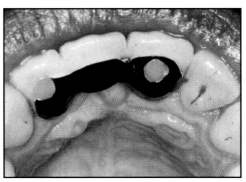
Fig. 20b A palatal view of the same bridge. The composite restorations on the palatal aspect of the 2/1 cover the retaining screws to the underlying implant abutments

Implant retained prostheses
An implant retained restoration is shown in figure 20.

Advantages
- Fixed or removeable
- Independent of natural teeth — can provide fixed restoration where no abutment teeth exist
- Immune to dental caries
- High level of predictability
- Good maintenance of supporting bone

Disadvantages
- Dependent upon presence of adequate bone quantity and quality
- Involves surgical procedure(s)
- Highly operator/ technique dependent
- High initial expense and lengthy treatment time
- Moderate maintenance requirements especially for removeable or extensive fixed prostheses

Treatment choices

In situations where all types of prosthesis are possible the final choice may rest with the patient, and is largely dependent upon their expectations/desires, financial budget and willingness to undergo treatment. It is important that the patient's expectations are realistic and achievable. However, some factors may dictate that a certain type of restoration is not feasible or is undesirable. This can best be illustrated by considering a number of case studies (see Case A to Case C).

Conclusion

The patient should be presented with the treatment alternatives and an indication of their respective advantages and disadvantages in their particular case. The treatment plans should be outlined in writing and an estimate of the relative costs given. Complex treatment plans require more detailed descriptions and a projected timetable for completion and costings. It is important to ensure that the patient understands the proposals and is given the opportunity to clarify any matters. A written consent to the agreed treatment plan is advisable.

Case A

Figure 21 shows a young female (aged 17 years) who has developmentally missing lateral incisors. While the removable prosthesis (Fig. 21b) provides reasonable appearance and function, it is understandable that a fixed alternative is desired by the patient. The space available for replacement of the missing teeth is narrow (about 4mm), thereby preventing placement of an implant, even if a narrow version is used. The patient has already undergone extensive orthodontic treatment and is unwilling to undergo more to create sufficient space. The adjacent abutment teeth are perfectly healthy and extensive preparation to provide a conventional bridge is contraindicated. Therefore the only fixed restoration that is feasible and desirable is a resin bonded bridge.

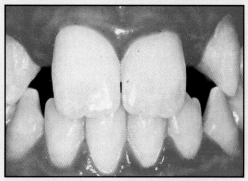

Fig. 21a This young individual has missing upper lateral incisors. Orthodontic treatment has provided only enough space for very small replacement teeth

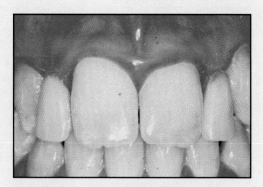

Fig. 21b The same patient is wearing a removable partial denture

Case B

Figure 22 illustrates a young female (aged 35 years) who lost four anterior teeth in an accident. The edentulous span is wide and the abutment teeth not ideal. The edentulous ridge form is good and a labial flange is not required for aesthetics or lip support. The present removeable prosthesis (fig. 22b) provides good aesthetics with a natural looking spaced dentition. She requests a fixed prosthesis. A diagnostic set up which eliminates the diastemas by increasing the number of prosthetic teeth is shown in fig. 22c). This setup would be required for a conventional fixed bridge but was unacceptable to the patient as she wanted to maintain the appearance of a spaced dentition. She therefore has two choices — a removeable prosthesis or four individual single tooth implants.

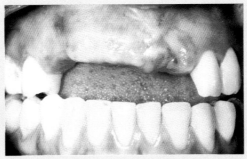

Figure 22a A large anterior endentulous space following traumatic loss of teeth

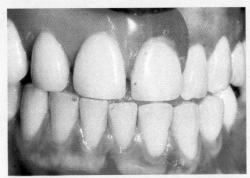

Fig. 22b The patient wearing a removable partial denture bearing four teeth with spaces between them

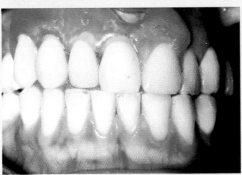

Fig. 22c The same patient with a diagnostic set-up placing five teeth in the gap and no spaces

Case C

Figure 23 shows a patient with a single missing anterior tooth. The adjacent teeth are crowned. In situations where the abutment crowns have a good prognosis, a conventional bridge would be the obvious choice. However, if the abutment teeth are supported by post crowns, they may be considered to have a questionable prognosis as bridge supports and an alternative replacement should be considered such as a single tooth implant.

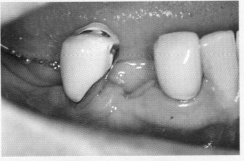

Fig. 23 A patient with a single missing upper incisor tooth. The adjacent teeth are crowned and have a good prognosis. Replacement of the missing tooth with a conventional bridge would be straightforward

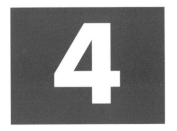

Treatment planning for implant restorations

Peter Floyd,[1] Richard Palmer,[2] and Vincent Barrett,[3]

Treatment planning for the provision of an implant retained restoration is essentially the same as that for the conventional restoration, except it also has to consider the provision of an adequate number, type, position and distribution of implants. It therefore involves a surgical phase of treatment (Part 6) and a time delay for the process of osseointegration to take place. The treatment plan should begin with a clear idea of the end result which should fulfil the functional and aesthetic needs of the patient. It is important that these goals are realistic, predictable and readily maintainable.

Types of implant restoration

Before considering the more detailed aspects of planning the following types of implant retained restoration are described:
- Fixed bridges
- Overdentures
- Single tooth restorations.

Fixed bridges

Implant retained fixed bridges range from limited span bridges to complete arch restorations for the edentulous jaw. There are two basic bridge designs, the original type as described by Branemark which was a cast metal bar with acrylic teeth and 'gumwork' attached to a number of implants and resembled a denture on stilts (fig. 1), and the more modern aesthetic approach where it resembles conventional

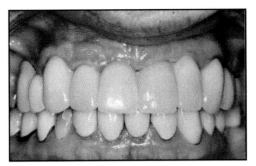

Fig. 2 An implant supported maxillary bridge opposing a crowned natural dentition. Maxillary bridges usually require a more aesthetic approach and the design of bridge gives the impression that the teeth are emerging from the gum. The bridge design in figure 1 would not be suitable in this case

bridgework with implants placed so that the prosthetic teeth appear to emerge from the natural soft tissues (fig. 2). These two designs will be considered in more detail.

The original Branemark 'bone anchored bridge' is the design on which many of the long-term success reports are based. It was largely used in the mandible and required the placement of five to six implants between the mental foramina. A cast metal framework is cantilevered distally, generally to a distance of about 12 mm but determined by the size of the bar and the maximum antero-posterior distance between implant centres.

In the mandibular arch, prosthetic stability has been reported for 99% of fixed prostheses over a 15-year period. However, lack of facial support and cheek biting can present appearance and functional limitations, especially in patients with more advanced bone resorption. Fixed prostheses in the mandible opposing a complete denture may also cause more bone loss in the opposing jaw than a mandibular overdenture. More frequent maxillary denture relines and potential for retention problems have been noted.

Although maxillary prosthetic survival rates of 92% have been reported over a 15-year period, more complications are encountered. Phonetic problems are the most frequent complaint. Spaces between the bridge and the underlying soft tissues result in breaks in the palatal contour and speech disruption. Oral hygiene may be compromised if acrylic flanges are extended over abutments and soft tissue

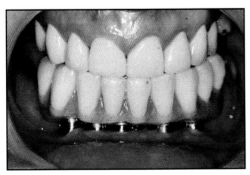

Fig. 1 The upper crowned natural teeth oppose a full-arch implant-supported bridge in the lower jaw. The bridge is similar in design and concept to that described by Branemark. Titanium abutments protrude a few millimetres through the mucosa and a space separates the bridge superstructure from the underlying mucosa. The prosthetic teeth are acrylic and have 'gumwork' in much the same fashion as a complete denture. This bridge is very rigid and is not removable by the patient

Treatment planning may be facilitated by determining the desired end result which meets the needs of the patient, and then planning in reverse order to achieve this goal.

In this part, we will discuss:
- Types of implant restoration
- Planning considerations
- Provisional restorations
- Treatment order

[1]Part-time Lecturer, Guy's Kings and St Thomas' Medical and Dental School, London SE1 9RT and Specialist in Periodontics, 4 Queen Anne Street, London W1 [2]Professor of Implant Dentistry and Periodontology, Guy's Kings and St Thomas' Medical and Dental School, London SE1 9RT, [3]Private Practitioner, 38 Devonshire St, London W1

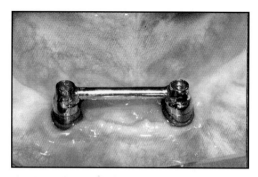

Fig. 3a Two mandibular implants joined together by a bar to support an overdenture

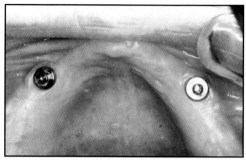

Fig. 3c Two individual implants with ball abutments used to support a maxillary overdenture. This solution is commonly used in the lower jaw but in the upper jaw the provision of more implants joined together by a bar is preferred

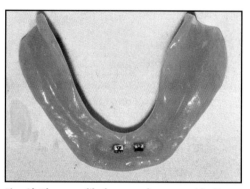

Fig. 3b The mandibular overdenture with clips in an anterior hollow which attach to the bar

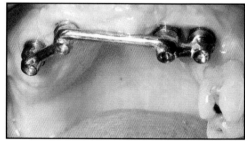

Fig. 3d Four maxillary implants joined together with a bar to support an overdenture

> **Type of implant restoration**
> - Fixed bridges
> - Overdentures
> - Single tooth restorations

hyperplasia may occur. Although the situation can be improved by placing a removable gingival veneer, they are complex and technically demanding restorations. The appearance can be very good but in patients with less ridge resorption or a high smile line, there is a greater likelihood of aesthetic problems.

Modern bridges usually have a cast metal framework extending beneath the soft tissue to connect to the implant abutments. The prosthesis is similar in design to a conventional fixed bridge prosthesis constructed on natural teeth and can be cemented or screw retained. In favourable circumstances, with minimal bone resorption, it is possible to achieve optimal aesthetics. Conversely when there has been substantial loss of bone, or when soft tissue replacement is required, it may be impossible to achieve the desired aesthetic result with this type of restoration. Where there is considerable labial resorption, the prosthetic teeth become progressively long, with large spaces apparent interproximally. In patients with a high lip line, the result is aesthetically unacceptable and the large spaces also compromise speech.

The intermaxillary relationship affects the design and use of these bridges. In restoring the maxillary arch in patients with an orthognathic jaw relationship (Angles Class 1), a ridge lap of the crown is not usually necessary. In situations where there is a severe space limitation, and ridge lap pontics are required for aesthetics, it is best to avoid implants in the incisor region.

Patients with a Class III malocclusion and more than minimal bone resorption may not be suitable for this type of maxillary fixed restoration. Cantilevering a fixed prosthesis more than one abutment diameter posteriorly and two abutments anteriorly is ill advised if the high bending moments during occlusal load are to be prevented. Patients with advanced bone loss are not usually suitable for these restorations because of the unfavourable biomechanics and inadequate facial and lip support.

Bone grafting may be necessary to avoid this problem (Part 8) or an alternative restoration chosen, such as an overdenture or patient detachable bridgework. In the latter design a cast metal bar is attached to an equivalent number of implants used for fixed bridgework. A superstructure bearing the prosthetic teeth and a labial flange can be removed by the patient for daily oral hygiene. The restoration is implant supported and although the teeth and labial flange are detachable there is a high level of 'security'. The restoration is difficult to manufacture, requiring a high level of precision with retention of the removable section of the prosthesis dependent on the accuracy of fit onto the milled bar.

Overdentures
These are patient removable complete dentures retained usually by implants joined with a straight round bar or with 'ball' attachments

(fig. 3). In the mandible the classic overdenture design is based on two implants placed in the mandibular canine regions and connected together by a bar which should be parallel to a line drawn between the mandibular condyles. The implants greatly improve retention and stability of the denture. Support for the denture is improved anteriorly but the posterior saddles are mucosal supported. In severely resorbed mandibles continued loss of bone has been reported in the molar areas. These overdentures may be also be retained by individual stud attachments with a high degree of success. In the maxilla, the failure rate is much higher, probably due to the poorer bone quality in the maxilla and high mechanical forces. It is usually recommended to provide at least four implants joined rigidly together with a bar (fig. 3d). Maxillary overdentures are more often opposed by a fixed dentition than mandibular overdentures and higher occlusal forces on the implants could be generated.

Single tooth restorations

Single tooth restorations are individual free-standing units not connected to other teeth or implants (fig. 4). They are similar to conventional single crowns and are normally cemented to prefabricated or customised abutments. Cantilever units are not normally recommended, and if two adjacent teeth are missing the requirement is for placement of two implants. If more than two adjacent teeth are missing, for example four incisor teeth, the decision has to be made whether to restore the space with four single units or a fixed bridge using fewer implants. The latter option is the one most often used because space is not normally available to provide an implant per tooth (see later section on implant spacing).

High success rates have been reported for single tooth restorations, particularly those replacing anterior teeth. Replacement of single molars is more problematic because of the size discrepancy between implant and tooth and the

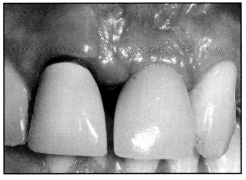

Fig. 4a The upper right central incisor has been replaced with an implant supported crown. This is often referred to as a single tooth implant. In comparison, the conventionally crowned upper left central incisor is not very aesthetic

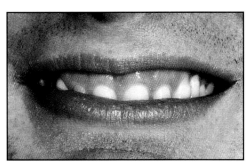

Fig. 5. A patient smiling who has a high lip line. A large area of gingivae is revealed which places high aesthetic demands if any of the anterior teeth require replacement

high occlusal loads. Therefore, wider diameter (5–6 mm) or two standard diameter implants may be used if space and finances allow.

Planning considerations

For simplicity, it will be assumed that treatment options other than implant retained restorations have been considered (Part 3) and there are no contra-indications. Planning begins with an assessment of the aesthetic and functional requirements, and proceeds to more detailed planning with intra-oral examination, diagnostic set-ups, appropriate radiographic examination (Part 5), and

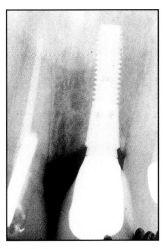

Fig. 4b A periapical radiograph of the single tooth implant in fig. 4a. The adjacent tooth has a post crown which would not have provided a suitable bridge abutment and the midline diastema would have precluded this option

Planning considerations
- Functional and aesthetic considerations
- Evaluation of the endentulous ridge
- Study casts and diagnostic set-ups
- Implant numbers and spacing

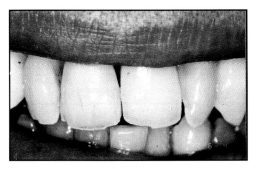

Fig. 6a This smile line does not have great aesthetic demands and it is difficult to determine which tooth has been replaced with a prosthesis

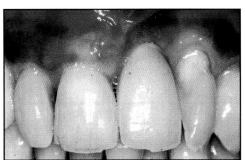

Fig. 6b An intra-oral view of the same individual revealing the implant retained crown at the upper left central incisor. The patient was happy to have a restoration which did not have a gingival margin at a level more consistent with the other teeth. This would have required preoperative grafting

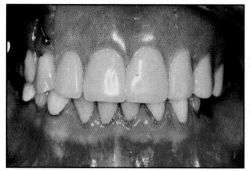

Fig. 7a A female patient with the maxillary anterior teeth replaced with an acrylic removable partial denture which has a labial flange. The patient requested an implant supported bridge and did not want a denture

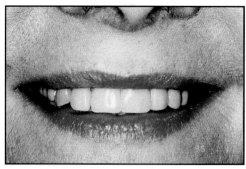

Fig. 7c The patient smiling with the original denture complete with labial flange

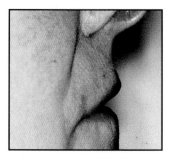

Fig. 7e Lip support in profile with the original denture

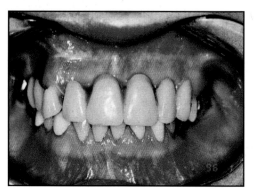

Fig. 7b The diagnostic set-up. Denture teeth have been set-up in a ridge lap fashion without a labial flange

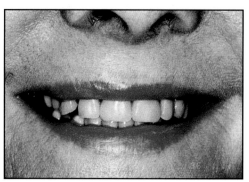

Fig. 7d The patient smiling with the diagnostic set-up. There is less lip support without the labial flange

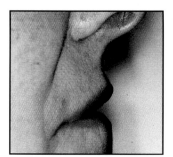

Fig. 7f Lip support in profile with the diagnostic set-up. Although there is less lip support the patient is satisfied with the appearance. Therefore it is possible to consider a fixed bridge reconstruction without additional lip support

construction of provisional restorations and surgical guides.

Functional and aesthetic considerations

Reduced or insufficient function is a common complaint for patients who have removable dentures or who have lost many molar teeth. Function of an otherwise adequate denture may be improved by providing implants to aid stability and retention. The alternative treatment is to replace the denture with a fixed bridge. The overdenture may be the treatment of choice where:

- The patient does not have a psychological problem with dentures and is quite happy to wear a removable restoration
- There is considerable resorption of the jaws allowing few implants to be placed
- The opposing jaw is restored with a satisfactory denture or the opposing teeth may be compromised by the occlusal forces generated by a fixed implant supported restoration.

The fixed bridge may be the treatment of choice where:

- There is a good dentition in the opposing jaw which may de-stabilise the denture. This is a particular problem where a natural dentition in the maxilla opposes an edentulous mandible (fig. 1).
- Patients have such a strong gag reflex that

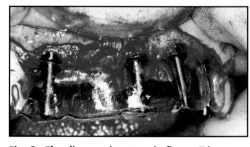

Fig. 8a The diagnostic set-up in figure 7 is transferred to a surgical guide to help the surgeon with positioning and angulation of implants. This figure shows a blowdown transparent stent and guide markers placed in the prepared implant sites

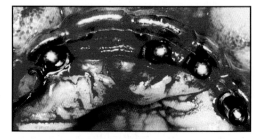

Fig. 8b The same stent and guides from an occlusal view showing the indicator guides behind the planned labial faces of the individual teeth which are to be replaced

they cannot tolerate a removable prosthesis
• Resorption of the jaws is not too advanced thereby allowing placement of an adequate number of implants, and the prosthetic replacement of large amounts of soft and hard tissue is not required.

A shortened dental arch extending to the first molar or second premolar should always be considered. Providing there are sufficient well distributed implants in the anterior part of the jaw, a distal cantilever extension can be used, thereby avoiding placement of implants in more difficult anatomical locations. Patients who request replacement of missing molar teeth need sufficient bone above the inferior dental canal or below the maxillary sinus floor to allow implants of sufficient length to withstand high occlusal forces. For example, replacement of the first and second molars would require a minimum of three standard implants joined together with a fixed bridge. The occlusion should be carefully assessed, particularly in all excursive movements. It may be helpful to examine the occlusion with the existing prosthesis or the provisional prosthesis to assess the type of loading to which the implant restoration will be subjected.

Aesthetic considerations may assume great importance in some patients. The coverage of the anterior teeth (and gingivae) by the lips during normal function and smiling should be carefully assessed (figs 5 and 6). An anterior restoration should also provide adequate lip support. The appearance of the planned restoration can be judged by providing a diagnostic set up or a provisional restoration (fig. 7). They may also serve extremely well as a model for the surgical stent or guide to assist in the optimal placement of the implants (fig. 8), and also as a transitional restoration during the treatment programme. Ideally, the patient should be examined with and without their current or provisional prosthesis to assess facial contours, lip support, tooth position and how much of the prosthesis is revealed during function.

Evaluation of the edentulous ridge

The height, width and contour of the ridge can be visually assessed and carefully palpated (fig. 9). The presence of concavities/depressions (particularly on the labial aspects) are usually readily detected. However, accurate assessment of the underlying bone width is difficult, especially where the overlying tissue is fibrous. This occurs on the palate where the tissue may be very thick and can result in a very false impression of the bone profile. Clinical techniques such as ridge mapping may help. The area under investigation is given local anaesthesia and the thickness of the soft tissue measured by puncturing it to the bone using either a graduated periodontal probe

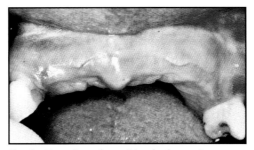

Fig. 9a The edentulous ridge in the patient shown in Figure 8. There is good ridge height and plenty of attached keratinised tissue

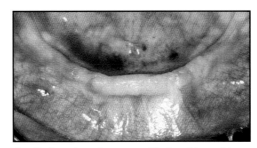

Fig. 9b An edentulous mandibular ridge with moderate to severe resorption. There is a small zone of attached keratinised mucosa

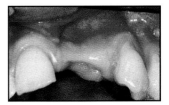

Fig. 9c A small edentulous area in the anterior maxilla. Traumatic loss of the teeth has resulted in considerable resorption and there is a marked concavity in the central incisor space

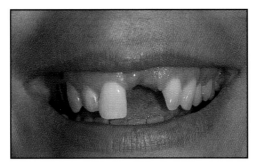

Fig. 10a A maxillary central incisor space. The ridge width appears good, but the thickness of the soft tissue may be deceptive

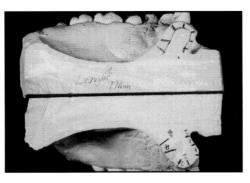

Fig. 10b A cast of the same patient which has been sectioned through the central incisor space. The bone contour has been mapped out on the cast by transferring clinical measurements of soft tissue thickness taken with a graduated probe after anaethetising the area

dental implants

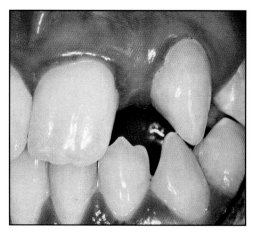

Fig. 11 A lateral incisor space which is narrow. The adjacent roots converge and therefore it would be impossible to place an implant without damaging the roots

or specially designed callipers. The information is transferred to a cast of the jaw which is sectioned through the ridge (fig. 10). This method gives a better indication of bone profile than simple palpation but is still prone to error. Whenever evaluation of the bone width and contour is critical, radiographic assessment is advised (Part 5).

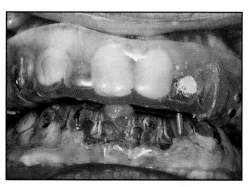

Fig. 12a A blow-down stent with radio-opaque markers placed at sites of interest

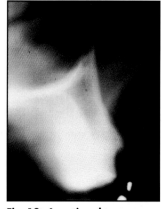

Fig. 12c A sectional tomogram through a marked site showing the marker and the ridge profile

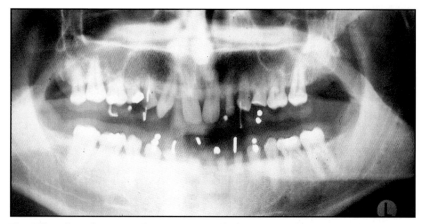

Fig. 12b A dental panoramic tomogram with the stent in place

The angulation of the ridge and its relationship to the opposing dentition is also important. The distance between the edentulous ridge and the opposing dentition should be measured to ensure that there is adequate room for the restorative components. Proclined ridge forms will tend to lead to proclined placement of the implants which could affect aesthetics and loading. Large horizontal discrepancies between the jaws, for example the pseudo class III jaw relationship following extensive maxillary resorption are not suitable for treatment with fixed bridges.

The clinical examination of the ridge also allows assessment of the soft tissue thickness which is important for the attainment of good aesthetics. Keratinised tissue which is attached to the edentulous ridge will also generally provide a better peri-implant soft tissue than non-keratinised mobile mucosa (Part 2). The length of the edentulous ridge can be measured to give an indication of the possible number of implants that could be accommodated. However, this also requires reference to radiographs to allow a correlation with available bone volume and the diagnostic set-up for the proposed tooth location. In edentulous ridges bound by teeth, the available space will also be affected by angulation of adjacent tooth roots, which may be palpated or assessed radiographically (fig. 11).

Study casts and diagnostic set-ups
Study casts, preferably articulated, allow detailed measurements of many of the factors considered in the previous section. The proposed replacement teeth can be positioned on the casts by the technician using either denture teeth or teeth carved in wax. The former have the advantage that they can be converted into a temporary restoration which can be evaluated in the mouth by the clinician and patient (fig. 7). The diagnostic set-up therefore determines the number and position of the teeth to be replaced and their occlusal relationship with the opposing dentition.

Once the diagnostic set-up has been approved it can be used to construct a stent or guide for radiographic imaging (fig. 12 and see Part 5) and surgical placement of the implants (fig. 8 and see Part 6). The stent/guide can be positioned on the original cast and with reference to the radiographs, the clinician can decide upon the optimum location, number, and type of implants.

Implant numbers and spacing
There are a few general guidelines as to the number of implants that are required in different situations (Table 1).

The more teeth which require replacement the greater the variation, especially when molar teeth are also considered. For example, four

Table 1	Implant requirements	
Fixed restorations:		
Anterior teeth	*Suggested number of implants required*	
One missing tooth	1	
Two missing teeth	2	
Three missing teeth	2 or 3	
Four missing teeth	2, 3 or 4	
Molar teeth		
One missing tooth	1 or 2	
Two missing teeth	2 or 3	
Full arch bridges		
Edentulous maxilla	at least 6	
Edentulous mandible	at least 4/5	
Overdentures		
Edentulous maxilla	at least 4 joined	
Edentulous mandible	2 joined or separate	

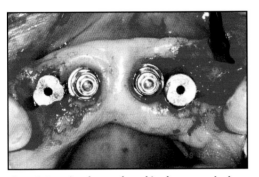

Fig. 13 Four implants placed in the upper incisor region. The implants in the central incisor sites have good spacing between them but the space between these and the adjacent lateral sites is too small. The implant components nearly touch and there is insufficient room for normal interdental tissue

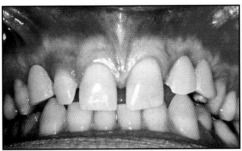

Fig. 14a A young man who has a number of developmentally missing anterior teeth which are replaced with a removable denture. There is spacing between the natural teeth

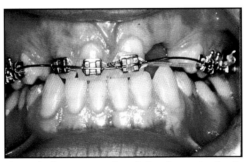

Fig. 14b The same patient following orthodontic treatment to close the anterior spaces and provide more room in the edentulous zones for adequate implant spacing, and better aesthetics

missing lower incisors could be replaced quite readily with two implants supporting a four unit bridge. Four missing upper incisors could be replaced with a bridge supported by three implants, but four implants would be required in a spaced dentition.

Two missing molar teeth would require three standard implants, or alternatively two wider diameter implants. Implants with different diameters can be chosen according to the tooth they are replacing. For example, most systems have a standard implant of about 4 mm in diameter that can be used in most situations. However, replacement of single upper lateral incisors, or lower incisors, may require narrower diameter implants (eg 3.25 mm) whereas a molar tooth may be more satisfactory replaced with an implant of 5 to 6 mm diameter.

It is a great mistake to attempt to place too many implants in a given space (fig. 13) and, if necessary, orthodontic treatment should be used to optimise spacing (fig. 14). Spacing is required to provide:
- An adequate width of bone and soft tissue between implants and adjacent teeth
- For the prosthetic components not to impact on each other
- For the patient to be able to clean the prosthesis effectively.

Implants placed next to natural teeth should allow an absolute minimum of 1 mm of intervening bone and preferably 2 mm. It is advisable to allow a little more spacing between implant heads, ideally 3 mm and no less than 2 mm. This is because in many systems the abutments are larger than the implant heads, and the restoration is often designed so that it increases in diameter to establish a good emergence profile.

With all these factors competing for space it is easy to see how the soft tissue and oral hygiene may be compromised if implants are placed too close together.

It should be noted that the above guidelines take no account of the differing implant diameters which are available. In many cases, manufacturer's recommend minimal centre-to-centre spacing of the implants, which is dependent upon their diameter and the minimum intervening tissue requirements described above.

The bone volume which can accommodate the proposed diameter and length of implant has to be determined radiographically. Implants should be selected to ensure optimum fixation, but seldom are implants longer than 15 mm required. In many instances the clinician is limited by the need to avoid damage to important anatomical structures, such as the inferior dental nerve. The assessment of length should allow an adequate safety margin, particularly as many drills are designed to prepare the implant site slightly longer than the chosen implant.

Provisional restorations

In the majority of treatment plans the provisional restoration is an essential component. It helps to establish the design of the final reconstruction and is used by the patient throughout the treatment stages. The following provisonal restorations are used:
- Complete denture
- Partial denture
- Adhesive bridgework
- Fixed bridgework.

Complete dentures are used as a provisional restoration for edentulous patients. There is a period (1–2 weeks) following surgical placement of implants when the dentures must not be worn. This avoids early transmucosal loading of the implants and allows adequate reduction of post surgical oedema to take place, facilitating proper adaptation of the denture. In general bone grafting and ridge augmentation procedures should not be carried out unless the denture can be left out for a considerable period after surgery.

Partial dentures can be used in anterior and posterior saddles and the same constraints apply as to full dentures (fig. 15). They are simple and inexpensive to construct. Acrylic dentures allow easy adjustment to accommodate any changes in tissue profile following implant placement and the transmucosal abutments when they are fitted.

Adhesive bridgework is most commonly used as a provisional restoration in the replacement of single teeth or small spans in anterior regions. A single tooth replacement is normally retained by a single adjacent retainer, whereas the replacement of multiple teeth requires

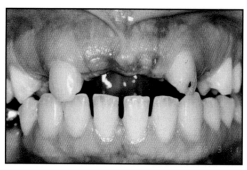

Fig. 15a Two implants have been placed in the central incisor sites

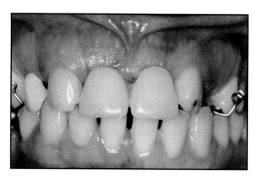

Fig. 15b A removable partial denture provides a satisfactory provisional restoration. It is important not to load the implants immediately after placement and therefore the denture should not be worn for 1 week, and in many cases 2 weeks

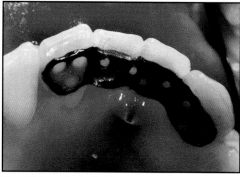

Fig. 16 A Rochette bridge used as a provisional restoration. The head of an implant can be seen beneath the mucosa

more abutments. Provisional retainers should be easily removable and, therefore, the Rochette rather than Maryland design is recommended (fig. 16).

Fixed bridgework retained by full coverage restorations may be the treatment of choice, particularly for patients having extensive treatment who are not prepared to undergo a period of time without a fixed restoration. This assumes the presence of a sufficient number of teeth to support the provisional or transitional bridge. It also enables ridge augmentation procedures to be carried out without the risk of transmucosal loading and the associated micromovement affecting the healing. The bridgework may have to remain in place some considerable time with frequent removal and replacement. Abutment teeth must be adequately prepared to allow for the casting of a metal framework of sufficient strength and rigidity and for the acylic/composite. Allowance should be made for the fact that the bridge will have to be modified following abutment connection.

Treatment order

Deciding on the treatment order may be very straightforward in some circumstances and in others extremely difficult, particularly for those cases involving transitional restorations.

A traditional plan may include the points listed in Table 2.

Conclusion

Treatment planning for implant restorations may at first appear complicated. It is imperative to consider all treatment options with the patient, and during detailed planning it may become apparent that an alternative solution is preferred. In all cases the implant treatment should be part of an overall plan to ensure health of any remaining teeth. Once the goal or end point has been established it should be possible to work back to formulate the treatment sequence. The cost of the proposed treatment plan is also of great relevance. The greater the number of implants placed, the higher will be the cost and this may therefore place limits on treatment options.

Table 2	Traditional plan

- Examination — clinical and initial radiographic
- Diagnostic set-up, provisional restoration and specialised radiographs if required
- Discussion of treatment options and decision on final restoration
- Completion of any necessary dental treatment including: extraction of hopeless teeth; periodontal treatment; restorative treatment, new restorations and/or endodontics as required
- Construction of provisional or transitional restorations if required
- Construction of surgical guide or stent
- Surgical placement of implants
- Allowing adequate time for osseointegration
- Prosthodontic phase.

Radiographic techniques

Peter Floyd,[1] Paul Palmer,[2] and Richard Palmer,[3]

Standard dental radiographs allow the clinician to make an initial assessment of the bone levels available for implant treatment, but as 2-dimensional images they give no indication of bone width. In combination with clinical examination they may provide enough information to plan treatment without resorting to more complex imaging techniques. Tomographic examinations can give cross-sectional and 3-dimensional images. In addition to providing information about bone quantity they also provide some indication of the bone quality available, notably the thickness of the cortices as well as an approximation of the density of the cancellous bone.

A standard classification of bone quantity and quality has been devised and is useful to describe the degree of alveolar resorption present (fig. 1), although the quality is often a subjective assessment and is more easily classified when surgery is performed. Radiographs are also used during treatment and provide an

assessment of osseointegration and long-term maintenance.

Screening

A screening radiograph should give the clinician an indication of:

- The overall status of teeth and supporting bone
- Those sites where it is possible to place implants using a straight-forward protocol
- Those sites where it is unlikely that implants can be placed without using complex procedures such as grafting
- Those sites where it is inadvisable to recommend implants
- Anatomical anomalies or pathological lesions.

In most instances the Dental Panoramic Tomograph (DPT) is the radiograph of choice (fig. 2). They provide an image within a predefined focal trough of both upper and lower jaws and as such give a reasonable approxima-

> **Radiographic examination is a central part of implant treatment from the planning phase to the long-term evaluation of treatment success.**

In this part, we will discuss:
- Screening
- Evaluation and planning
- Perioperative and follow-up radiographs

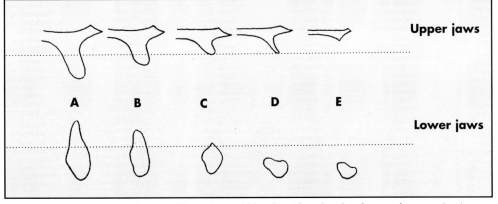

Fig. 1a Ridge resorption in the maxilla and mandible. The ridge shortly after tooth extraction is described as morphology A through progressive degrees of resorption to grossly atrophic E

Fig. 1 A classification of ridge resorption described by Lekholm and Zarb (1985).
Redrawn from Lekholm U, Zarb G. Patient selection and preparation in *Tissue Integrated Prostheses*. Branemark P I, Zarb G A, Albrektsson T (eds). pp199–210. Quintessence, 1985

Fig. 1b Bone quality is on a four point scale: Type 1 is mainly cortical, Type 2 is a dense cortex and cancellous space, Type 3 is a thinner cortex and less dense cancellous bone, Type 4 has a very thin cortex and sparse bone trabeculae in the medullary space

[1]*Part-time Lecturer, Guy's Kings and St Thomas' Medical and Dental School, London SE1 9RT and Specialist in Periodontics, 4 Queen Anne Street, London W1* [2]*Part-time Demonstrator, Guy's and St Thomas' Hospital Trust, London SE1 9RT and Specialist in Periodontics, 21 Wimpole Street, London W1* [3]*Professor of Implant Dentistry and Periodontology, Guy's Kings and St Thomas' Medical and Dental School, London SE1 9RT*

tion of bone height, the position of the inferior dental neurovascular bundle, the size and position of the maxillary antra and any pathological conditions which may be present. They are therefore an ideal view for initial treatment planning and for providing patient information as they present the image in a way that many patients are able to understand. These are narrow beam rotational tomographs which use two or more centres of rotation to produce an image of the dental arches. Some areas may not be imaged particularly well, but this can be minimised by ensuring that the patient is positioned correctly in the machine and that the appropriate programme is selected. The radiation dosage of a DPT is approximately 0.007 to 0.014 mSv which is less than a full mouth series of periapical radiographs where each periapical accounts for about 0.001 to 0.008 mSv. They provide more information about associated anatomical structures than periapical radiographs but with less fine detail of the teeth. It should be remembered that all DPT's are magnified images [at around ×1.3]. Distortion also occurs in the antero-posterior dimension reducing their usefulness when planning implant spacing and numbers.

The information provided by a DPT can usefully be supplemented using other standard extra-oral and intraoral radiographs. For example, the lateral cephalogram can give more detail of the morphology of both jaws close to the midline, and this can be useful when planning overdenture treatment (fig. 3). Standard occlusal views may also aid in assessing the bone morphology in the lower jaw. Should further information be required following the screening examination, then the appropriate tomographic examination is made.

Radiography for single tooth replacement or small bridges in individuals with little bone loss can normally be accomplished by intra-oral radiographs taken with a long cone paralleling technique. However it must be remembered that an overall evaluation of the mouth should be made for a full assessment of treatment needs. Image quality is of the utmost importance and it should be ensured that all relevant anatomical structures are shown on the image being used and that any allowances for distortion of the image are made. This is particularly important when assessing available bone height above the inferior dental canal and when working close to other important anatomical structures.

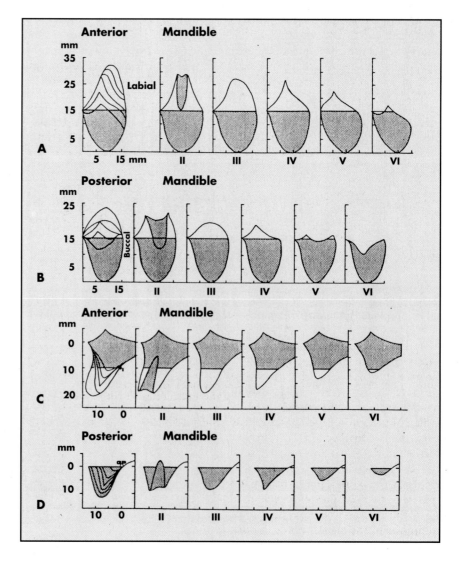

Fig. 1c Classification of jaw resorption as described by Cawood and Howell (1991):
(A) classification of anterior mandible (anterior to mental foramen)
(B) classification of posterior mandible (posterior to mental foramen)
(C) classification of anterior maxilla
(D) classification of posterior maxilla. Reproduced by kind permission of Munksgaard International Publishers Ltd, Copenhagen, Denmark. From Cawood J I, Howell R A, *Int J Oral and Maxillofac Surg* 1991; **20**: 75

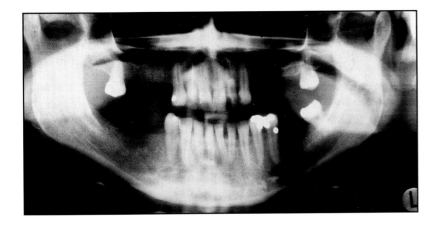

Fig. 2a A dental panoramic tomogram of a partially dentate individual who wished to be treated with implant retained prostheses. This initial screening radiograph suggests that there is sufficient bone height above the inferior dental canal in the lower right jaw and below the maxillary sinuses. More detailed information of this patient is presented in results of a CT scan in figure 5

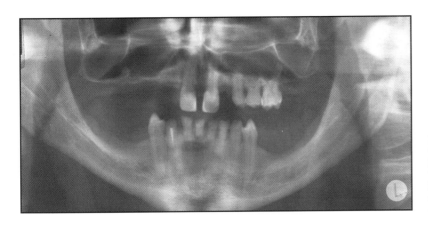

Fig. 2b A dental panoramic tomogram of a patient with oligodontia. It clearly shows very little bone height in the right maxillary edentulous region. This area is only treatable following extensive bone grafting. The only significant bone mass in the upper jaw is in the premaxilla

Computerised digital radiovisiography is becoming more commonplace and can provide an alternative medium to produce an image. As the detectors are solid state the doses used can be greatly reduced. Additionally, manipulation of the digitally derived image may provide further information about relative bone densities, particularly when assessing peri-implant bone density changes by subtraction radiography. It is likely that their application in implant dentistry will become more widespread.

Evaluation and planning

Radiographic stents

In order to optimise the information provided by more advanced radiographic techniques, it is necessary to provide information about the planned final restoration. A stent which mimics the desired tooth setup is constructed and radiographic markers usually made of gutta percha or another radio-opaque material placed within it (fig. 4a). Alternatively, if the patient has a suitable acrylic denture, radiographic markers may be placed within occlusal or palatal cavities cut in the acrylic teeth. The denture can also be replicated in clear acrylic to provide the radiographic stent. The radiopaque marker or rod can be placed in the position and angulation of the planned prosthetic set-up. Thus for a screw retained prosthesis the marker would indicate the access hole for the screw retaining the

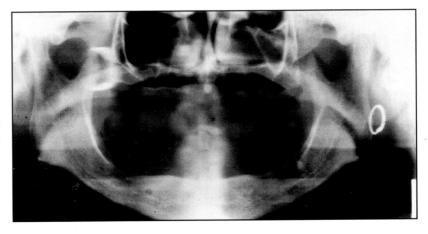

Fig.3a A dental panoramic tomogram of an edentulous individual with good bone height in the mandible, particularly in the symphyseal region (Class C). There is extensive resorption in the maxilla (Class E). The mandible is treatable with implants and the maxilla would require extensive grafting

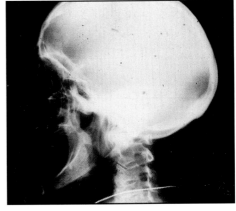

Fig. 3b A lateral skull view demonstrates the ridge profile of both upper and lower jaws in the midline

restoration. Alternatively the relation of the bone ridge to the proposed tooth set-up can be shown by painting the labial surface of the stent with a radiopaque varnish (fig. 4b). The choice of radiographic marker is important in that it should be visible on the radiographic image but not interfere with the scan. When using Computerised Tomography (CT), metal markers should be avoided as they can produce scattering on the image (see later). Stents are particularly useful in the edentulous patient as they also serve to stabilise the position of the jaws while the radiographs are being taken. When using CT for edentulous patients this is most desirable because of the long exposure time. The stent can also provide the radiographer with a true occlusal plane from which to orientate the axial scans.

Simpler types of stent involve placing radiopaque markers eg ball bearings of various diameters or twisted wire shapes into a baseplate and are designed to help determine mesiodistal location.

Computerised tomography (CT scan)

CT scans provide the clinician with the most detailed images currently available, but given their cost and high radiation dose their use is often limited to more complex cases such as full arch maxillary reconstructions, bilateral posterior mandible imaging or to assess whether patients require extensive grafting procedures (fig. 5). CT uses x-rays to produce sectional images as in conventional tomography. High resolution images are achieved by initially scanning in an axial plane keeping the sections thin and by making the scans contiguous or overlapping. The large number of sections in a high resolution scan of a jaw approximates to a radiation dose of 3 mSv. New generation helical CT scanners are faster and have significantly lower radiation dose. The scans should be limited to the area of interest and avoid radiosensitive tissues such as the eyes. In place of conventional film the radiation is detected by highly sensitive crystal or gas detectors which is then converted to digital data. This data can then be stored and manipulated by computer software to produce a grey-scale image. The software then allows multiplane sections to be reconstituted, the quality of which are dependent on the original scan section thickness and integers between successive sections.

Images can be produced as:
- Standard radiographic negative images on large sheets
- Positive images on photographic paper often in book form
- Images for viewing on a computer monitor.

Whatever the presentation format, it is of great importance to align the scan properly. The patient's head is aligned in the scanner

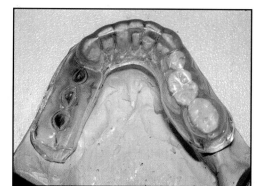

Fig. 4a A simple radiographic stent constructed on a cast of the mandible. This stent is a blowdown plastic with radioopaque markers at the sites of planned implant placement, to guide the radiographer to the areas of interest for sectional tomography

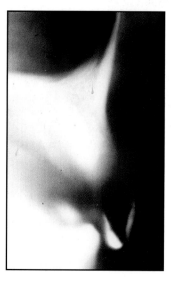

Fig. 4b A sectional tomograph through a maxillary ridge with the patient wearing a radiographic stent in which the outline of the proposed teeth has been imaged by applying a radioopaque varnish. This allows an estimation of the position and angulation of the implant in relation to the prosthesis by the clinicians planning the restoration and the surgery

Fig. 5 Computerised axial tomography of the jaws of the same patient illustrated in figure 2

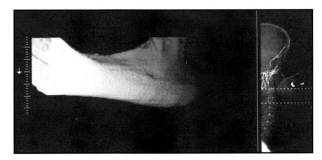

Fig. 5a This shows a 3-dimensional reconstruction of the mandible and a lateral scout view showing the plane of the sections parallel to the occusal plane

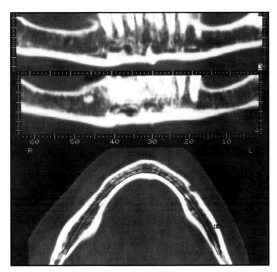

Fig. 5b The lower part of the figure shows a horizontal section through the mandible which is in the same plane as the original scan slices. The computerised data from these slices is reformatted to produce all of the other images in figure 5. The upper part of the figure shows two slices in the same plane as a DPT but at different depths through the mandible

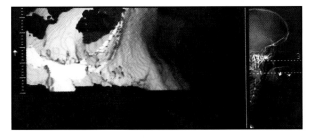

Fig. 5d A 3-dimensional reconstruction of the right maxilla

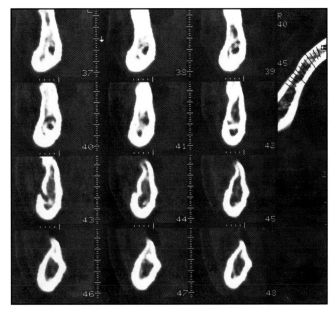

Fig. 5c Cross sectional images of the right mandible. The location of the cross sections is shown on the horizontal section in the top right corner of the figure.The mental foramen is clearly shown in section 43 and the inferior dental canal can be traced in sections distal to this (higher numbers) and the incisive branch anteriorly. The sections give an indication of the cortical thickness and density of trabeculation within the central part of the jaw

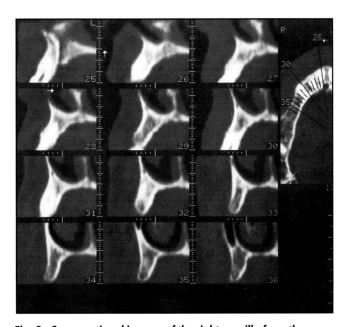

Fig. 5e Cross-sectional images of the right maxilla from the midline (section 25 showing the incisive canal) to the premolar area. The nasal cavity is visible on most of the sections. The last section 36 shows the anterior part of the maxillary sinus (laterally) and the nasal cavity with the inferior turbinate. The location of the cross sections is shown on the horizontal section in the top right corner of the figure

with light markers, and a scout view obtained which gives an image similar to a lateral skull film (fig. 5a). The radiation dose of this scout view is low and can be repeated if the alignment is incorrect. Generally the mandible is scanned with slices parallel to the occlusal plane and the maxilla using the same plane or one parallel to the floor of the nose. Deviation from this alignment will result in the cross-sectional slices not being in the same direction as the proposed implant placement (See radiographic stents).

Figure 5 illustrates the reformatted images which can be produced including:

dental implants

Fig. 6. This shows radiographic images taken on a Scan Ora

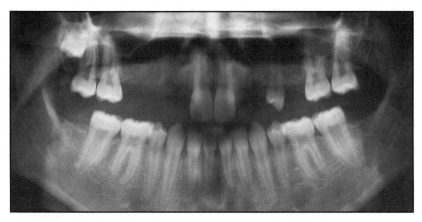

Fig. 6a The high quality DPT image is produced at a magnification of x1.7. This shows a patient with failure of development of multiple permanent teeth in the maxilla

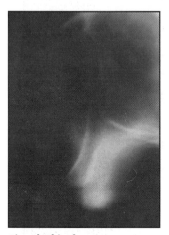

Fig. 6b This shows a cross-sectional image of the maxillary ridge in the same individual. The height and width determinations must take account of the magnification

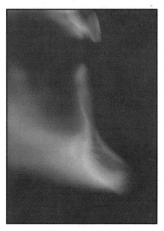

Fig. 6c A Scan Ora section through the anterior mandible of the patient whose DPT is shown in figure 2b. The cross section shows a retained deciduous incisor and a very thin bone profile apical to this. The thickness improves at the chin

- Sections in the same plane as the original slices (the raw data)(fig. 5b)
- Cross-sectional images of the jaw at right angles to the original plane of slice, numbered consecutively and radially around the arch. These are the most useful images (fig. 5c and 5e)
- Images in the same plane as a conventional DPT, but at different depths (fig. 5b).
- 3-dimensional reconstructions of the surface morphology of the jaw (fig. 5a and 5d).

Heavy metals will produce a scatter-like interference pattern if they are present in the slice under examination and the interference will therefore appear in all the generated sectional images. Extensive interference may render a CT scan unreadable and can be produced by large posts in root canals or heavily restored teeth where the plane of examination passes through such a tooth as well as an area of critical interest.

In some instances therefore either a compromise has to be made in the direction of scanning or a different method of examination chosen (eg scan ora, see later). Consideration should also be given to removing the offending metal prior to examination if appropriate in the overall treatment plan.

The various scan images can be measured for selection of implant length and diameter. Although the nominal magnification of the images is 1:1 some machines and cameras produce images where the magnification may vary. A scale is usually incorporated alongside the various groups of images and the real magnification can be determined from this. A correction factor can then be applied to measurements taken directly from the films.

In contrast to hard copies of the scans, one of the advantages of the computer-based image software programs (eg Simplant) is that it is possible to produce images of implants (and their restorative components) which can then be 'placed' within the CT scan. This enables the clinician to evaluate the relationships between the proposed implants and ridge morphology, anatomic features and adjacent teeth. When used in conjunction with a radiographic stent the possibilty of reproducing the orientation envisaged at the planning stage is greatly increased.

Scan Ora

Scanora is an example of a new generation of sophisticated tomographic devices most similar to conventional DPT machines, but with facilities to generate high quality sectional images (fig. 6). In contrast to CT scanning where the sectional images are software generated, the Scan Ora produces a tomographic image directly onto film. It uses complex broad beam spiral tomography and is able to scan in multiple planes. The scans are computer controlled with automatic execution but still rely heavily on good patient positioning and experience in using the machine. The patient's head is carefully aligned within the device and this position recorded with skin markers and light beams. A DPT image is produced from which the sites which require sectional tomographic data are determined (fig. 6a). The patient is repositioned in exactly the same alignment and the appropriate tomographic programme selected for the chosen region of the jaw.

The Scan Ora magnification is ×1.3 or ×1.7 for routine DPTs but is ×1.7 for all sectional images. Tomographic sections are normally 2 mm or 4 mm in thickness (figs 6b and 6c). As with all tomograms the image produced includes adjacent structures which are not within the focal trough which therefore appear blurred and out of focus. Because the scan sections are thicker and fewer the overall patient dose is much less than a CT scan. The amount of detailed information provided is considerably less than a CT scan but is usually sufficient for all but the most complex cases.

In order to facilitate planning using images at different magnifications, transparent overlays depicting implants of various lengths and diameters at the corresponding magnifications can be superimposed directly on the radiograph. These provide a simple method of assessing implant sites and implant placement at different angulations.

Perioperative and follow-up radiographs

Intra-oral radiographs may be useful at the time of implant placement allowing visualisation of drills or direction indicators and their relation to adjacent teeth or anatomical structures. Radiovisiography is useful as it produces an instant image at a lower radiation dose. At second stage surgery radiographs may be required to ensure full seating of abutments when direct visualisation has not been possible at the time of surgery (See Part 4).

During the prosthetic phase it is essential to ensure full seating of components and frameworks (fig. 7). This may not be possible by direct vision because of the soft tissues, and radiographs provide the only method of checking fit. It is essential that radiographs are taken at 90° to the long axis of the implant under examination and it is therefore recommended to use long cone parallel radiographs. Only a relatively small deviation from the correct angulation may make the radiograph unreadable. Correct angulation is easy to check when using threaded implants as the thread profile is clearly seen when the x-ray is taken at 90°(fig. 7).

Baseline radiographs to show crestal bone levels and the state of the peri-implant bone should be taken as part of normal documentation at the time of fitting the final prosthesis. These should be repeated on an annual basis for the first 2 or 3 years to establish that the bone levels are stable. It should be remembered that some initial bone loss will occur during the first year of function with some implants but that a steady state should then be established thereafter. The interval between radiographs may be extended if the bone appears stable over the first few years of function (See Part 10).

Many of the problems which arise during treatment or once the prosthesis is in function are most readily diagnosed using standard intra-oral views (figs 8 and 9), these include:
- Burnt bone syndrome
- Bone loss
- Component loosening
- Screw breakage
- Implant fracture
- Adjacent endodontic lesions
- Loss of integration.

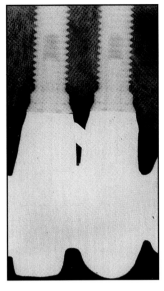

Fig. 7 A periapical radiograph of the restoration framework try-in. Th implant thread profiles are clearly visible which indicates that the film was taken with a good paralleling technique. This enables the clinician to check that the abutments are correctly seated on the implants, the framework fits the abutments and that the bone levels at this stage are close to the top of the implant

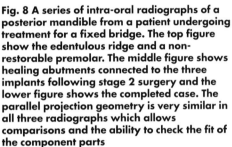

Fig. 8 A series of intra-oral radiographs of a posterior mandible from a patient undergoing treatment for a fixed bridge. The top figure show the edentulous ridge and a non-restorable premolar. The middle figure shows healing abutments connected to the three implants following stage 2 surgery and the lower figure shows the completed case. The parallel projection geometry is very similar in all three radiographs which allows comparisons and the ability to check the fit of the component parts

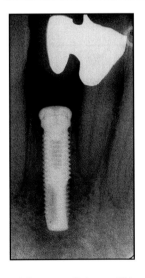

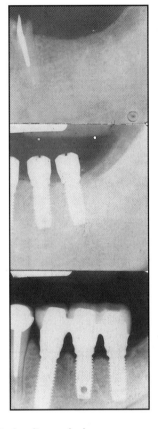

Fig. 9. This periapical radiograph shows an implant which was placed approximately 4 weeks previously. An adhesive bridge provides the provisional restoration. The patient experienced discomfort and the radiograph shows an apical radiolucency around the implant. Bone resorption has occurred because of damage to the bone at implant placement. This is caused by failure to cool the bone during the drilling operation and is referred to as burnt bone syndrome

These conditions will be dealt with more fully in Part 10, Complications and Maintenance.

Conclusion

Radiographs play an important part in the successful planning and execution of implant treatment. It is important to have an understanding of the different techniques available and their appropriate application. They are an important part of the patients records and as such constitute a significant proportion of the medico-legal documentation of the patient. It is the responsibility of the clinician to ensure that radiographs are appropriate, readable and are retained and repeated at accepted intervals throughout treatment and follow-up.

Basic implant surgery

Richard Palmer,[1] **Paul Palmer,**[2] **and Peter Floyd,**[3]

Successful implant surgery is largely dependent upon good planning and meticulous technique. The former requires an appreciation of the restorative requirements and visualisation of the desired end result of treatment, whereas the latter requires adequate surgical training and experience of the selected implant system.

The essential pre-requisites before proceeding to implant surgery are:

- The patient should be medically fit to undergo the surgery. Placement of one or two implants is equivalent to relatively minor oral surgery whereas placement of five or six implants increases the magnitude significantly. The medical history should be checked with particular relevance to:

    Poorly controlled diabetes
    Blood dyscrasias
    Medications
    Irradiation to jaws
    Mucosal diseases
    Psychoses
    Substance abuse including tobacco and
        alcohol
    Need for antibiotic cover.

- The patient should understand the procedure and be warned of any complications. They should have agreed the treatment plan, treatment schedule, costings, and given their consent.
- The diagnostic set-up surgical stent and relevant radiographs should be available.
- The surgeon should have a clear idea of the number, size and planned location of the implants. They should be trained in the procedure and able to cope with any unforseen circumstances.

Operative requirements

Most implant surgery can be carried out in a well equipped dental surgery. Ideally the surgery should be designed to permit surgical procedures under good aseptic conditions. The following should be available:

- Good operating light
- Good high volume suction
- A dental chair which can be adjusted by foot controls or by a third party
- A surgical drilling unit which can deliver relatively high speeds (up to 3000 rpm) and low drilling speeds (down to about 10 rpm) with good control of torque
- A purpose designed irrigation system for

keeping bone cool during the drilling process
- The appropriate surgical instrumentation for the implant system being used and the surgical procedure
- Sterile drapes, gowns, gloves, suction tubing etc.
- The appropriate number and design of implants planned plus an adequate stock to meet unexpected eventualities during surgery
- The surgical stent
- The complete radiographs including tomographs
- A trained assistant
- A third person to act as a runner between the sterile and non-sterile environment.

Anaesthesia and analgesia

Most implant surgery can be carried out under local anaesthesia, although some patients will require sedation or general anaesthesia. The surgical time will vary greatly between different operators and cases. Short cases, for example under 1 hour for placement of one or two implants do not usually present problems with anaesthesia. Complex cases may take 2 or 3 hours and it is essential to use regional block anaesthesia (infra-orbital, palatal, inferior dental) and to supplement this during the procedure. Local infiltrations are also administered as they improve the anaesthesia and more importantly control haemorrhage. Sedation is recommended for operations of long duration eg more than 90 minutes. It is a good idea to give analgesics, such as ibuprofen or paracetamol, immediately prior to surgery.

Sterile technique

Every effort should be made to conduct implant surgery under sterile operating conditions. Chlorhexidine 0.2% is used as a pre-operative mouthwash and skin preparation circumorally. The patient is draped as for other oral surgical procedures, and drill leads should be autoclaved or covered with sterile tubing. Light handles should be autoclaved or covered with sterile aluminium foil. It is convenient to use sterile disposable suction tubing and stents. The instrument tray and any other surfaces which are to be used are covered in sterile drapes.

Surgical techniques for implant installation

Surgical installation of implants requires good visualisation of the bone ridge profile and

Implant surgery protocols differ slightly with individual systems. However, basic surgical principles are required to ensure successful osseointegration of the implant in the correct location which allows good aesthetics and loading.

In this part, we will discuss:
- Operative requirements
- Surgical techniques for implant installation
- Post-operative care
- Surgery for abutment connection

[1]*Professor of Implant Dentistry and Periodontology, Guy's Kings and St Thomas' Medical and Dental School, London SE1 9RT* [2]*Part-time Demonstrator, Guy's and St Thomas' Hospital Trust, London SE1 9RT and Specialist in Periodontics, 21 Wimpole Street, London W1* [3]*Part-time Lecturer, Guy's Kings and St Thomas' Medical and Dental School, London SE1 9RT and Specialist in Periodontics, 4 Queen Anne Street, London W1*

dental implants

meticulous preparation of the bone site to accept the implant (figs 1, 2 and 3).

Anatomical considerations

The implant surgeon should be fully conversant with all anatomical structures that they are likely to encounter or that will affect implant placement, including:
- *In the maxilla*
  - Air sinuses
  - Nasopalatine canal
  - Floor of nose and nasal spine
  - Palatine and pterygoid vessels
- *In the mandible*
  - Sublingual vessels
  - Mental nerve
  - Inferior dental nerve
  - Incisive branch of inferior dental nerve
  - Genial tubercles
- *Teeth*
  - Position, length and angulation of roots adjacent to implant sites
- *Available bone*
  - Ridge morphology
  - Bone density
    - Cortical
    - Medullary
  - Localised deformities
    - tooth sockets
    - residual cysts/granulomata.

Flap design

There are many different flap designs for implant surgery. In practically all situations a mid-crestal incision can be employed. Access and elevation of the flaps can usually be improved by the additional use of vertical relieving incisions (fig. 1a,b) Relieving incisions close to adjacent teeth can be made to include the elevation of the (interdental) papilla, but some surgeons prefer to avoid raising this in case future aesthetics are compromised. Care should be taken to ensure that incision lines are not placed over structures such as the mental nerve and the palatine arteries. All incisions are made through periosteum down to bone.

Full thickness mucoperiosteal flaps are raised carefully to expose the entire extent of the edentulous ridge where the implants are to be placed (fig. 1b). The flaps should be elevated sufficiently far apically to reveal any bone concavities, especially at sites where perforation might occur. Important anatomical structures in the area of operation which might be damaged, such as the mental nerve, should be identified and protected.

Surgical preparation of the bone

It is essential not to allow the bone to be heated above 47°C during preparation of the site as this will cause bone cell death and prevent osseointegration. This problem may be avoided by:
- Using sharp drills
- Employing an incremental drilling procedure with increasing diameter drills
- Avoidance of excessive speed (no more than 3,000 rpm) and pressure on the drills — ensuring that the drill is withdrawn from the site frequently to allow the bone swarf to clear. This is particularly important in dense/hard bone
- Using copious sterile saline irrigation. This can be delivered from a sterile infusion bag in a pressure cuff or a peristaltic pump. The drills can be adequately cooled by spraying the external surface of the drill. However, some systems use internally irrigated drills.

A typical sequence of drilling and implant insertion is shown in figure 1. Preparation of the sites commences with penetration of the outer cortex with a small round bur followed by twist drills of increasing sizes The drills are marked to indicate the corresponding lengths of implants. The spacing and angulation of the implant sites are checked carefully with direction indicators throughout the drilling sequence, in relation to the stent and the opposing jaw/dentition. The angulations should be checked from different viewpoints (eg buccal and occlusal) as it is very easy to make errors when viewing from a single aspect.

Implant placement

The ideal siting and orientation of the implant is dictated by the restorative requirements, but this may have to be modified by the existing ridge morphology and adjacent anatomical structures. Following elevation of the flaps the surgical stent should be tried in. In partially dentate cases the stent should be stabilised on adjacent teeth and provide guidance of where the planned labial faces, occlusal surfaces or cingulae of the teeth to be replaced are to be located. An example of a suitable stent is shown in figure 1c. In edentulous cases it is far more difficult to provide a stable stent as it will have to rely upon a mucosal fit in areas where the mucoperiosteum has not been raised.

Ideally an implant should be placed such that:
- It is within bone along its entire length. Exposure of limited areas of implant surface associated with bone defects such as dehiscences or fenestrations may be acceptable, but larger ones may require augmentation (Part 8).
- It does not damage adjacent structures such as teeth, nerves, nasal or sinus cavities. It is acceptable to engage the nasal or sinus floor with a small degree of penetration (eg 1 to 2 mm). An adequate safety margin of about 2 mm above the inferior dental canal is recommended.
- It is located directly apical to the tooth it is replacing and not in an embrasure space.
- The angulation of the implant is consistent with the design of the restoration. This is particularly important with screw retained restorations where it is desirable to have the

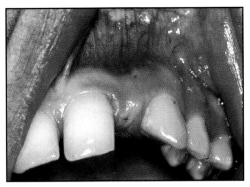

Fig. 1a The pre-operative view of the upper left lateral incisor space

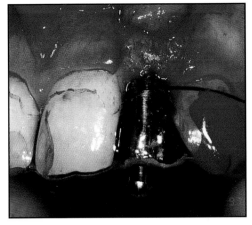

Fig. 1d A guide or indicator post is placed in the site to check on the position and angulation of the implant. Small adjustments can be made at this stage

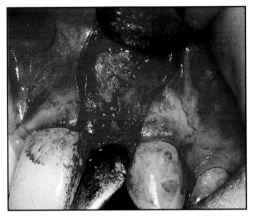

Fig. 1b A full thickness mucoperiosteal flap has been elevated to completely expose the alveolar ridge to determine its shape and whether any concavities are present. The flap has vertical labial relieving incisions, a crestal incision mesio-distally and has included elevation of the papillae to give good access to the narrow edentulous space

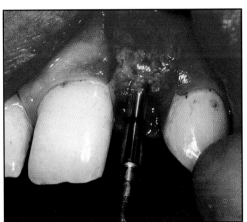

Fig. 1e The site is enlarged by a pilot drill. This has a non-cutting end of the same diameter as the previous twist drill and a wider cutting portion. It should therefore maintain the line of the previous drill

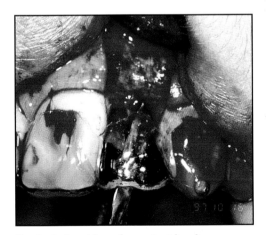

Fig. 1c A clear blow-down stent has been placed over the adjacent teeth and provides the surgeon with the position of the labial face and gingival margin of the tooth which is to be replaced. The initial preparation of the implant site is with a round bur which readily penetrates the cortex, and this is followed by a twist drill (illustrated) which determines the initial angulation and depth of the implant

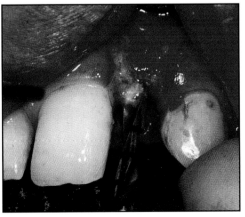

Fig. 1f The site is enlarged with the final twist drill which is slighlty narrower than the implant itself. The drill has marks on it corresponding to the available implant lengths. All drilling to this stage is carried out at moderate speeds (about 1,500 rpm) with copious saline irrigation

Fig. 1 This series of photos show a standard sequence of surgery for the placement of an individual implant (Nobel Biocare) in the upper lateral incisor space

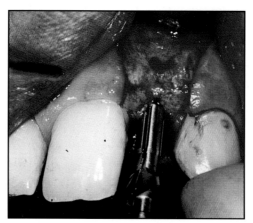

Fig. 1g The surface of the bone is countersunk to accept the head of the implant. The depth of countersinking is determined by the need to sink the head of the implant to allow a good emergence profile of the restoration. The head of the implant should therefore be about 2 to 3 mm apical to the labial cement-enamel junction on the adjacent teeth or apical to the planned gingival margin determined by the stent

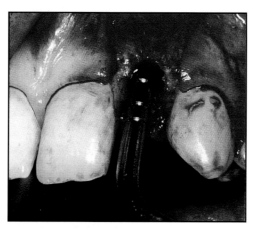

Fig. 1h The depth of the implant site is verified with a measuring guage

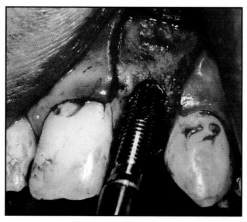

Fig. 1j A self tapping implant is inserted into the prepared site at slow speed and with irrigation

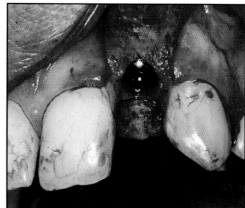

Fig. 1k A cover screw is placed on top of the implant

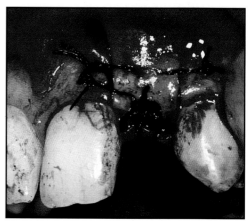

Fig. 1m The flap is closed with black silk sutures

restoration (fig. 2). However most systems allow convergence/divergence of up to 30° without the use of angled/customised abutments.

- The top of the implant is placed sufficiently far under the mucosa to allow a good emergence profile of the prosthesis. This is often achieved by countersinking the head of the implant (fig. 1g). For example, it is suggested that the top of a standard diameter implant (about 4 mm) when used to replace a single upper incisor tooth, should be 2 to 3 mm apical to the labial cement enamel junction of the adjacent natural tooth.
- There is sufficient vertical space above the implant head for the restorative components.
- The implant should be immobile at placement. A loose implant at this stage will fail to osseointegrate.
- Adequate bone is present between adjacent implants, and between implants and adjacent teeth (fig. 2). This should preferably be about 3 mm and never less than 1 mm. In some cases 1 mm of bone may be acceptable implant spacing, but the abutments may have a larger diameter and therefore prevent proper abutment seating, thereby complicating the restorative procedure. A distance of 3 mm will also allow better soft tissue adapta-

screw access hole in the middle of the occlusal surface or cingulum of the final restoration. Multiple implants are placed in a fairly parallel arrangement, to facilitate seating of the

tion and may allow the maintenance of an 'interdental papilla'.

The above requirements are not always easy to achieve and in many circumstances would be impossible without a properly designed stent produced from the diagnostic set up. Inevitably there are situations where a careful balance is needed between the ideal 'set up' and possible implant placement.

Implant insertion

The technique for insertion of the implant depends largely upon the system being used. In general the final bone preparation site diameter is slightly smaller than the implant. The size of the site can be adjusted according to bone quality or density. In poor quality bone the site can be made relatively smaller to produce compression of the surrounding bone on implant insertion which will improve the initial stability. In dense bone the site has to more closely match the size of the implant. In bone with relatively poor medullary quality, where initial stability may be difficult to achieve, it is often advisable to secure the implant at each end in cortical bone (bicortical stabilisation) providing anatomical structures, length of implants and ability to provide adequate cooling allow this. The implant is supplied in a sterile container, either already mounted on a special adapter or unmounted necessitating the use of an adapter from the implant surgical kit. In either case the implant should not touch anything (other than a sterile titanium surface) before its delivery to the prepared bone site. Screw shaped implants are either self tapped into the prepared site (fig. 1j and 2c) or inserted following tapping of the bone with a screw tap (fig. 3a). Cylindrical implants are either pushed or gently knocked into place. The installation of the implants should be done with the same care as the preparation of the site by maintaining the cooling irrigation and placing the implant at slow speeds. Screw shaped implants and tapping of sites are performed at speeds of less than 20 rpm. Following placement the head and inner screw thread of the implant is protected with a 'cover' or closure screw (fig. 1k and 3c).

The mucoperiosteal flaps are carefully closed with multiple sutures either to bury the implant completely (fig. 1m) or around the neck of the implant in non-submerged systems (fig. 3c). Silk sutures are satisfactory and others such as PTFE or resorbables (eg vicryl) are good alternatives.

Post-operative care

After implant surgery, patients should be warned to expect:
- Some swelling and possibly bruising
- Some discomfort which can usually be controlled with oral analgesics
- Some transitory disturbance in sensation if

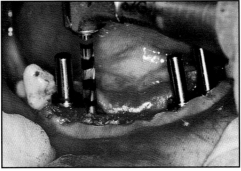

Fig. 2 This shows a short sequence of multiple implant placements (Astra implants) in a large edentulous space in the anterior mandible

Fig. 2a Flaps have been raised and four sites are being prepared. Direction indicators are inserted into the sites to allow the surgeon to verify the planned angle and in this case to keep them fairly parallel to one another. A stent was used in the initial positioning but has been removed to allow easier visualisation

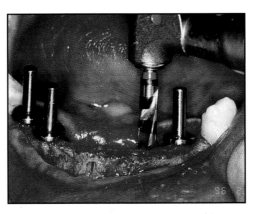

Fig. 2b This shows a later part of the procedure in which a twist drill is enlarging the sites further. The surgeon has been working sequentially from left to right with each of the drilling stages

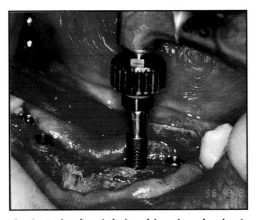

Fig. 2c An implant is being driven into the site. It is connected to a slowly rotating handpiece by an implant mount and handpiece connector

surgery has been close to a nerve.

They should be advised:
- In most circumstances, not to wear dentures over the surgical area for at least 1 week (possibly 2 weeks) to avoid loading the implants and the possibility of disrupting the sutures
- To use analgesics and ice packs to reduce swelling and pain

dental implants

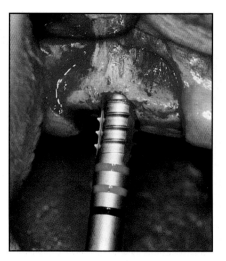

Fig. 3a The drilling sequence has been completed and a tap is being used to cut a thread in the bone. The coloured marks refer to the length of standard implants

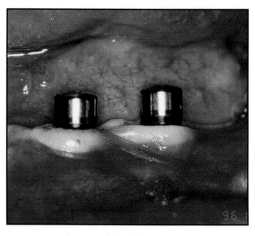

Fig. 4 Small incisions have been made in the mucosa overlying submerged implants to allow removal of cover screws and placement of healing abutments

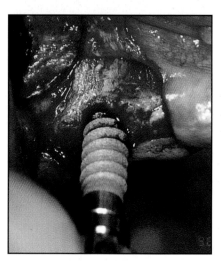

Fig. 3b The solid threaded implant is being screwed into the site using a hand ratchet. This is done slowly with irrigation

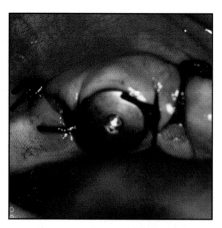

Fig. 3c A closure screw has been placed on top of the implant and the flaps sutured around the implant neck

- To keep the area clean by using chlorhexidine mouthwash 0.2% for 1 minute twice daily
- Not to smoke. This compromises healing of

soft tissue and bone and may increase the risk of implant failure. Ideally patients should stop smoking for some weeks before surgery and for as long as possible thereafter.

The need for systemic antibiotic cover should be considered. The original protocols recommended an antibiotic such as amoxicillin 250 mg 8 hourly for 5 to 7 days, unless the patient is allergic where a suitable alternative should be prescribed. Alternative regimes include administration of 3 grams of amoxycillin 1 hour before surgery, or 500 mg every 8 hours for 48 hours. Treatment plans which have used provisional bridges have an advantage in that they do not load the implant sites and can be refitted immediately after the surgery, providing some allowance has been made to accommodate some swelling. All patients should be seen after 1 week for review, suture removal and adjustment and refitting of dentures with adequate soft linings. In some cases the tissues will not be able to accept a denture for 2 weeks. This is most likely with surgery in the edentulous mandible and with surgical flap designs which affect the sulcus shape. Patients will require regular review and change of soft liners. In some cases there may be exposure of cover screws, but this has little effect on the success of the implant providing they are kept clean.

Surgery for abutment connection
(Second stage surgery)

In non-submerged systems (fig. 3), a second surgical stage is not required and abutments are simply exchanged for the closure screws after a period of about 3 months. In general, submerged implants placed in the mandible are exposed and loaded earlier than those in the maxilla (around 3 months compared with 6 months) because of differences in bone quality. Exposure of the implant at stage 2 surgery can be achieved with minimal flap reflection or

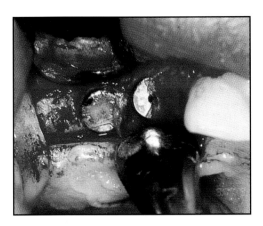

Fig. 5a A buccal flap has been raised to expose the cover screws attched to the heads of two implants. The crestal incision has been placed towards the palatal aspect so that the overlying keratinised tissue can be mobilised towards the buccal aspect

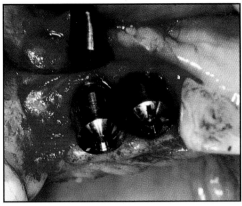

Fig. 5b The cover screws have been removed and healing abutments placed. These are simple titanium cylinders which should just protrude through the mucosa

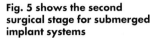

Fig. 5 shows the second surgical stage for submerged implant systems

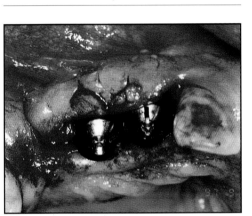

Fig. 5c The buccal flap is shaped with a scalpel to more acurately fit the healing abutments. The small pieces of tissue have been left attached rather than being removed as they can be rotated and positioned between the implant to optimise coverage of the bone

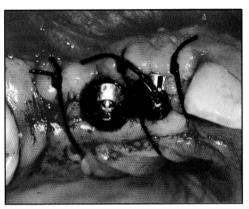

Fig. 5d The flaps have been sutured so as to fit neatly around the healing abutments

sometimes making a very small incision over the implant just to allow removal of the cover screw and attachment of an abutment (fig. 4). In some cases bone grows over the cover screw and this necessitates greater soft tissue reflection to allow bone removal with hand instruments, burs or specially designed mills prior to abutment connection. Most systems employ specially designed healing abutments which allow good mucosal adaptation and healing before selection of the abutment for the final restoration. Ideally the healing abutment should protrude about 1 mm above the mucosa. It is important to check that the abutments are fully seated on the implant. This can be achieved during surgical exposure by direct vision and radiographically at later stages.

Handling of the soft tissue at abutment connection surgery should aim to preserve keratinised (and preferably attached) mucosa on the labial and lingual aspects (fig. 5). The position of the crestal exposing incision should serve to achieve this goal. For example, keratinised tissue overlying the implant or towards the palatal aspect can be repositioned to the buccal aspect. A number of techniques have been described to optimise soft tissue contours to produce well formed interdental tissues and aesthetic papillae (fig. 5c and 5d). An overlying prosthesis will need to be adjusted to accommodate the protruding abutment. Prostheses which are designed and made with this in mind help considerably. The patient should expect some post-operative discomfort and be advised to take analgesics. They should use chlorhexidine mouthwash until adequate oral hygiene can be re-established. The soft tissue healing will allow the restorative phase to commence in 3 to 4 weeks.

Conclusions

Implant surgery is highly technique sensitive and requires adequate training and an understanding of the restorative requirements of the proposed treatment. However, control of these factors can produce a highly predictable, aesthetic and long-lasting result. In instances where there is insufficient bone and or soft tissue to allow successful implant placement and subsequent restoration, grafting and augmentation procedures will be required, and these are dealt with in Part 8.

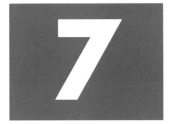

Basic restorative techniques

Leslie Howe,[1] Vincent Barrett,[2] and Paul Palmer,[3]

The restorative phase of treatment starts before the implants are placed. It is essential that a clear idea of the final result should be envisaged so that the dentist and patient can appreciate any limitations or compromises that may be needed. The restorative dentist will be responsible for the fabrication of any radiographic or surgical guides that may be required to help in the surgical positioning of the implant. Provisional restorations that maintain appearance and function during implant treatment are also the restorative dentists' responsibility.

The restorative dentist familiar with routine prosthodontic techniques will recognise many of the basic procedures involved in the restorative phase of implant treatment. There is much in common: thorough examination and treatment planning, diagnostic work-up that includes tooth selection, positioning and occlusal contacts, indirect techniques with crown and bridge impression materials, accurate jaw relation and occlusal records. However, implant supported restorations also require a mechanism for attaching the restoration to the implant and this component is termed the abutment. Its selection, placement and the recording of its position with adapted impression techniques is the main difference between conventional and implant prosthodontic techniques.

The standard restorative procedure for implant restorations allows the clinician to record accurate impressions of the abutment by using machine made copings. This is a significant advantage over tooth-borne restorations in that the copings guarantee marginal detail while the impression accurately relates the abutments to one another, any remaining teeth

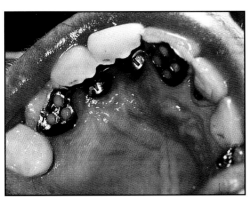

Fig. 1 Rochette bridge used as a provisional restoration

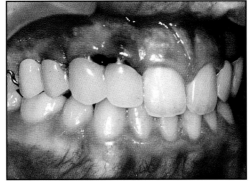

Fig. 2 A provisional partial acrylic denture needs to allow for adjustment when the healing abutments are placed

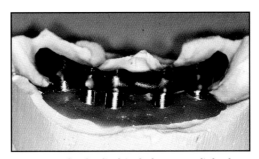

Fig. 3 Standard cylindrical abutments linked together with a composite resin bar ready for try in

and the soft tissue detail. Replicas of the abutments are then placed into the impression which is then cast in dental stone to provide a representation of the abutments on which machine made gold or ceramic cylinders are used to fabricate the restoration.

Provisional restorations

Before starting implant treatment a provisional or transitional restoration should be made that will be durable throughout what can sometimes be a lengthy course of treatment.

The requirements of a provisional restoration are that it should allow for the implant sites to be minimally loaded immediately after initial surgery. They should also be designed so that they are easily adapted following placement of healing abutments and subsequent implant restorative procedures. In its simplest form a provisional restoration may be a modification to an existing prosthesis but could also involve extensive fixed bridgework made with a metal framework/composite resin veneer.

Some restorative techniques for implant supported restorations will be familiar to dentists used to providing conventional crown and bridgework. The differences and principles involved when using implants are identified.

In this part, we will discuss:
- Provisional restorations
- Abutment selection
- Seating the abutment
- Impression taking
- Laboratory techniques
- Jaw relation registration
- Try-in appointment
- Framework try-in
- Restoration insertion
- Occlusion
- Follow-up appointment
- Overdentures

[1]Consultant in Restorative Dentistry, Guy's and St Thomas' Hospitals Trust, London SE1 9RT and Specialist in Restorative Dentistry and Prosthodontics, 21 Wimpole Street, London W1M 7AD; [2]Private Practitioner, 38 Devonshire Street, London W1; [3]Clinical Demonstrator in Periodontology, Guy's, Kings and St Thomas' Medical and Dental School, London SE1 9RT and Specialist in Periodontics, 21 Wimpole Street, London W1M 7AD

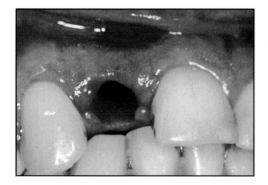

Fig. 4a An Astra single tooth implant with the healing abutment removed

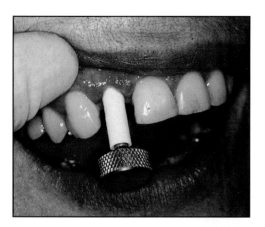

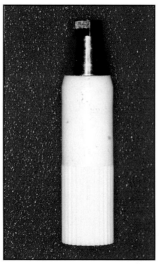

Fig. 4b Single tooth abutment attached to holder. Note the tapered abutment with antirotation shape at the base

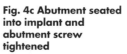

Fig. 4c Abutment seated into implant and abutment screw tightened

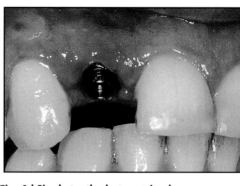

Fig. 4d Single tooth abutment in place

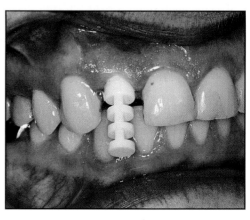

Fig. 4e Impression coping attached

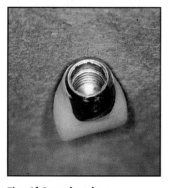

Fig. 4f Completed crown. Note the retentive shape which cannot rotate

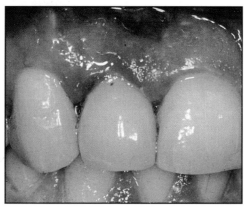

Fig. 4g Completed crown

For single teeth, consideration should be given to a resin bonded bridge designed so it can be relatively easily removed. A Rochette bridge with a perforated retainer is a good option (Fig. 1). Once again the pontic should be mainly acrylic to allow for later adjustment. Such a bridge can be easily removed and reinserted at the surgical stages, allowing the patient to remain dentate throughout treatment.

When the patient is edentulous, complete dentures should be made to allow adequate relief over the implant sites. Immediately following implant surgery a period of a week or more when dentures cannot be worn is strongly recommended and thereafter soft lining materials such as those for tissue conditioning are used to reline the denture base. The patient should be advised to avoid biting food directly over the surgical site. Removable partial dentures should be constructed with subsequent adjustments in mind which not only include the period following surgical implant placement but also after the healing abutment and final restorative abutment are in position (Fig. 2). If this is done with care a metal base removable partial denture can be made but often a simple acrylic denture is easier to adapt.

Sometimes it is not possible to adapt the provisional restoration after the abutments are placed and consideration should be given to making a provisional restoration on the implant abutments. While this may be seen as an inconvenient further step in treatment, provisional restorations can provide invaluable diagnostic information about tooth arrangement, position and shade for the definitive restoration.

Abutment selection

Abutments are components that attach to the implant head and are retained to the implant by an abutment screw that extends through the abutment into the body of the implant. The abutment extends through the gingiva into the oral cavity and it provides the support for the restoration.

The simplest abutment is a titanium parallel sided cylinder that extends from the implant head through into the oral cavity by 1–2 mm.

From the top of this cylinder, bridgework can be made linking the abutments together (Fig. 3). This traditional approach will produce the 'oil rig' style bridge that most readers will be familiar with. It is particularly useful for lower fixed bridges where appearance is not of paramount importance.

In recent years the number of abutments available for all implant systems has dramatically and confusingly increased. The main types are:

Single tooth abutments

These are designed to incorporate an anti-rotation device both at the junction of the abutment to the implant and also between the abutment and the restoration (Fig. 4). The final restoration can be cemented or screw retained, the cemented restoration being most popular as it is more aesthetic and the angulation of the implant is less important. Single tooth abutments are chosen so that the margin for the restoration is about 2 mm sub-gingival and machine cylinders for crown construction can be precious metal or porcelain, both having very high fit accuracy.

Fixed bridgework abutments

These abutments are designed to be linked by the restoration to each other and so do not require anti-rotation features between the abutment and the bridge (Fig. 5). The abutments are secured to the implant head in the normal way. The bridge end of the abutment is tapered to allow for different paths of insertion of the implants to be overcome by a fixed framework which is either retained by gold screws or conventional cementation. Angled abutments are available to overcome severe alignment problems between implants.

Overdenture abutments

Either ball attachments or magnets can be used which are incorporated into the abutment or several implants can be linked together with a bar onto which a denture can be retained by clips (Fig. 6). Abutments have to be selected dependent upon the available space within the denture.

Armed with the knowledge of which abutment type is to be used an appropriate length of abutment can be chosen. The healing abutment is unscrewed and the height of soft tissue from the rim of the implant head to the gingival margin measured with a periodontal probe. If possible and where necessary, the abutment is selected so that the margin for the restoration is placed 1–2 mm subgingivally.

Abutment selection
- Single tooth abutments
- Fixed bridgework abutments
- Overdenture abutments

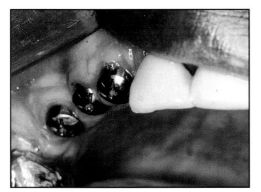

Fig. 5a Three Branemark implants ready to be restored. Healing abutments are in place

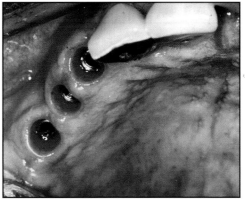

Fig. 5b Healing abutments removed. The head of the implant can be seen with a raised hexagon portion around the screw-hole which will act as positive location for the abutment

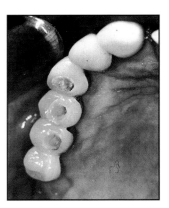

Fig. 5e Palatal view. The access holes for the screws have been restored with composite resin

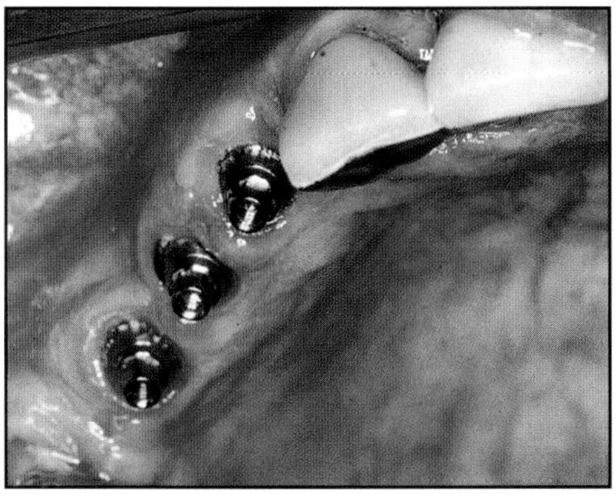

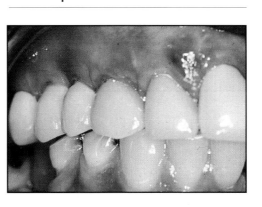

Fig. 5c Bridge abutments in place (Estheticones)

Fig. 5d Completed bridge (one extra pontic has been cantilevered distally)

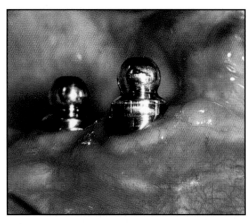

Fig. 6 Overdenture abutments

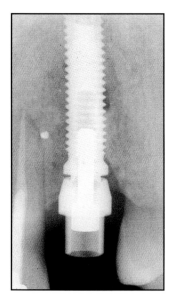

Fig. 7 Radiograph of incorrectly seated single tooth abutment

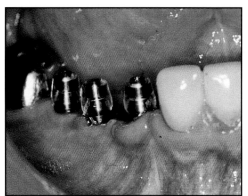

Fig. 8 Astra bridge abutments covered with clear plastic protection copings

Seating the abutment

Once the appropriate abutment has been selected it is then seated onto the implant head. It is essential that full seating is ensured and as the abutment-implant junction is commonly subgingival, checking with an intra-oral radiograph may be needed (Fig. 7). When full seating has been verified, the abutment screw can be tightened to the manufacturer's recommended level of force using a torque wrench. When the level of torque force needed is high it is advisable to hold the abutment with a counter-torque device.

Plastic healing caps are available to cover the abutments once they have been placed and the

provisional restoration will need to be adjusted to accommodate the additional components (Fig. 8). Alternatively the abutment can be removed at the end of each appointment and the healing abutment replaced onto the implant. In this situation final screw tightening is delayed until the final placement of the restoration.

Impression taking

The aim of an impression for implant restorations is to record the implant positions in a master working cast. Many techniques have been described and materials used in making impressions. While there is no consensus on any one way of making the impression, whichever method is used, it should be done with an understanding of the technique and the properties of the impression material. Impression materials should be resilient enough to be removed from undercuts without distortion and rigid enough to allow for accurate seating of components into the impression and to prevent movement of components during pouring of the impression in dental stone.

Primary impressions can be made with irreversible hydrocolloid (alginate) in a stock tray and for the definitive impression a stock tray

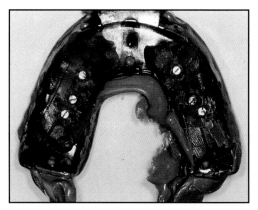

Fig. 9b Impression in a stock tray removed from mouth. The retaining screws are visible through the window in the tray to allow them to be unscrewed

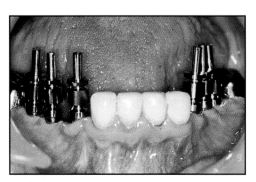

Fig. 9a Impression copings for 'pick up' impression

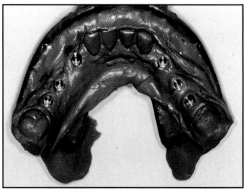

Fig. 9c From the fit surface the impression copings are checked for stability

will be adequate for single tooth implant impressions or short span bridges. For more extensive cases a custom tray is preferable for the final impression, not only to ensure an optimal thickness of impression material for dimensional stability, but also to record sulci and retromolar pad areas.

There are many choices of impression technique. The standard approach is an impression made of the implant abutment using a transfer impression coping.

There are two types of implant transfer impression coping: pick-up and re-seating copings.

The pick-up implant impression coping is used with a open faced impression tray. The tray allows access to a retaining screw that secures the impression coping to the implant. The retaining screw must extend 2–3 mm above the impression tray opening (Fig. 9). Impression material in injected around the impression copings first and then the tray is seated in the mouth. After the impression material has set and before removing the tray, the retaining screw is unscrewed leaving the pick-up impression coping inside the impression. The implant laboratory replica is then attached to the coping before pouring the impression with dental stone (Fig. 10). For a single tooth, the impression is made with a plastic push on coping that fits snugly over the abutment and can be picked up in a rubber base impression as above (Fig. 11).

The re-seating impression coping is used with a conventional impression tray and syringing technique and the coping remains in place on the implant after the impression material has set and the impression removed from the mouth (Fig. 12). The transfer coping is then unscrewed from the implant and attached to the laboratory replica outside the mouth and the coping/replica is re-inserted into the impression before pouring with dental stone. This technique is useful in clinical situations where there is limited space to allow for screwdrivers to undo the long retaining screws of the pick-up technique.

Laboratory techniques

Many of the laboratory techniques for implant restorations are essentially the same as for conventional prosthodontic treatment. Working casts are made using precise replicas of the abutments and machine-made gold cylinders that fit the abutments accurately can be incorporated into conventional framework wax-ups and then cast in a suitable precious gold alloy. Casts are normally made with a flexible silicone rubber gingival cuff, which is removable from the cast, allowing the dental technician to make sure that there is an accurate fit of the abutment/restoration in the subgingival region and to help visualise and create emergence crown con-

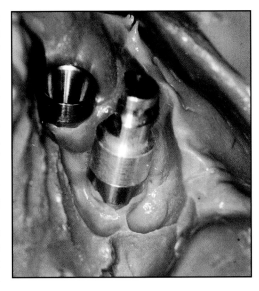

Fig. 10 The abutment replica is attached to the impression coping prior to making the cast

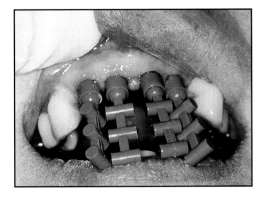

Fig. 11a Branemark single tooth impression copings seated for a 'pick up' impression

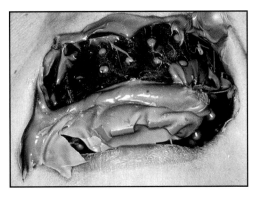

Fig. 11b The copings will be removed from the mouth in the impression

tours and profiles that are consistent with the gingival margin.

Implant supported bridges can either be made using conventional metal ceramic techniques or using denture teeth set in acrylic resin or using laboratory composite materials attached to a suitably designed metal framework. Choice of material will depend on a number of factors, not least restorations in the opposing dentition and any tendency towards parafunctional grinding habits.

Jaw relation registration

Conventional jaw relation records are made for single tooth and short span bridgework. The same principles for establishing occlusal plane, freeway space and recording the retruded position are applied to extensive bridgework or

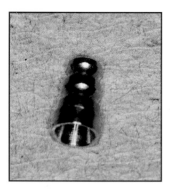

Fig. 12a Reseating impression coping. Note the ribbed design to allow for the coping to be accurately reseated in the impression

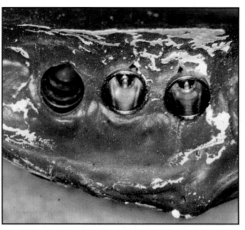

Fig. 12b Impression detail. The ribbed shape can be seen in the impression

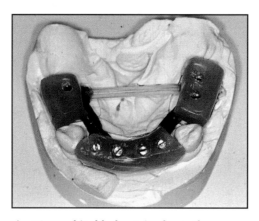

Fig. 13 Wax bite block retained onto the abutments ready to be tried in and trimmed

edentulous treatments with the advantage that bases for occlusal rims can be secured firmly to the abutments (Fig. 13).

The gold cylinders are fixed into a cold cured or light cured resin bar and a wax rim attached. This also allows the clinician to check the accuracy of the working cast and any misfit can be corrected by sectioning the acrylic bar and rejoining with an autopolymerising resin (Fig. 3).

Try-in appointment

From the records of the previous appointment the laboratory are able to fabricate a try-in using acrylic teeth set onto the resin bar or by waxing up the entire set-up (Fig. 14). This can then be used to check the appearance and occlusion as well as phonetics and cleansibility of the final restoration. It is best to check all of these features before the final framework casting is made for any longer span bridges. Single tooth restoration and short span bridges are normally produced directly from the impression stage and do not require try-in appointments.

Framework try-in

For long span bridges it is important that the final framework is tried in the mouth before the final fit appointment. It is desirable to have a perfect passive fit of the framework onto the abutments (Fig. 15). This is best checked by placing the framework in the mouth secured by only one retaining screw. It should seat fully with no obvious spring or discrepancy. This should be repeated using different abutments to ensure a perfect fit. Discrepancies in fit require sectioning of the bridge and repair with an autopolymerising resin to allow repouring of the master cast and soldering of the framework. If the framework is passive the remainder of the screws should be inserted and tightened sequentially to check that no tension is produced in the bridgework. This is usually indicated by discomfort to the patient. If the framework has been soldered it is important to repeat this appointment to check the fit once more.

Restoration insertion

If all other procedures have been performed correctly the fit appointment should be reasonably straightforward. However the application of acrylic or porcelain can produce stress within the framework which may effect fit, and the procedures for framework try-in should therefore be repeated to check the final fit. The occlusion and appearance need to be checked and the patient given appropriate oral hygiene instruction. The bridge screws can then be progressively tightened in sequence in an order that will not produce stress within the bridge.

Bridge screws are tightened to 10 NCm and provisional restorations are placed in the screw access holes with cotton wool or gutta percha protecting the screw heads.

Occlusion

For single tooth restorations or limited span bridges, occlusal contacts need to be examined in light and heavy contact. It should be remembered that the implant is in effect ankylosed and so will not move under occlusal contact when compared with a tooth. If the restoration was made so that it was in full contact under initial occlusal contact, then once pressure was applied the implant restoration would take the full load and possibly be overloaded. In initial occlusal contact therefore the implant restoration should be in enough contact to lightly mark occlusal indicator paper but should not hold shim stock. As pressure is exerted by the patient so the implant restoration can come to hold shim stock.

It is important that the restoration is not totally out of occlusion because the risk is that there may be uncontrolled overeruption of the opposing teeth resulting in a loss of occlusal stability and occlusal interferences.

In eccentric jaw movements the ideal is not to have contact on the implant retained restoration. Where possible, immediate dis-

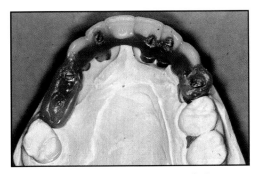

Fig. 14 Prior to casting the framework the cylinders have been linked together with a composite beam and the teeth waxed in to verify appearance and tooth position

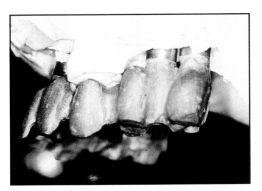

Fig. 15 The fit of the metal casting need to be verified both on the model and in the mouth

clusion on a natural canine is preferable. When anterior teeth/canines are involved in the restoration attempts should be made to provide occlusal contacts over multiple teeth and implants.

In the completely edentulous patients, implant retained dentures should follow conventional occlusal concepts of bilateral balanced or lingualised occlusion. For fixed full arch bridges the aim is simultaneous contact on anterior and posterior teeth in centric relation with anterior group function and multiple contacts in eccentric jaw movements (no canine guidance).

Follow-up appointment
At the follow-up visit the occlusion and oral hygiene should be checked. The temporary restorations over the screw holes are removed and the screws checked for tightness. Some loosening is acceptable at this stage and ¼ turn of the screw may be required to achieve full

seating of the screw. If more than ¼ is required it is possible that an error in fit or occlusion is present and will require adjustment. Once happy that the screws have remained tight, the access holes can be filled with the composite resin after covering the screw head with gutta percha. Accurate long cone periapical radiographs should be taken to confirm the final fit and record the marginal bone height for future comparison.

Overdentures
Complete overdentures retained by implants are made to conventional prosthodontic principles. As with tooth borne overdentures, the bases should be designed to allow intimate tissue contact over the maximum support area and peripheral extension to achieve a border seal. Excessive reduction of the base extension in an attempt to appease patients' wishes for less tissue coverage may lead to unfavourable loading of the implants.

The main feature of the implant abutments is to provide a retentive feature for the overdenture and to improve the stability of the denture base. These might include ball, magnet or clip attachments. The main difference between implant and tooth-borne dentures is the design of the support. Cantilever support may be used to a limited degree in implant retained overdentures with a bar and clip, but not normally in tooth borne restorations.

Jaw relation records should create a freeway space of 2–4 mm in the incisor region and tooth position that provides for an adequate lip support and even bilateral posterior occlusal contacts which allow for freedom in movement.

Conclusion
Attention to detail during the prosthetic phase of implant treatment can produce highly aesthetic restorations which will continue to function at a high level over many years. The treatment planning phase is essential to make sure that the prosthodontic treatment is kept as straightforward as possible. Many of the shortcomings of conventional dentistry are avoided because of the use of manufactured components. However failure to observe the basic rules of conventional and implant dentistry can lead to problems which may be difficult and expensive to overcome.

Implant surgery to overcome anatomical difficulties

Paul Palmer,[1] and Richard Palmer,[2]

The indications for employing corrective or reconstructive surgical techniques may be functional and/or aesthetic and may involve both hard and soft tissues. Sufficient bone must be present to allow placement of an implant of appropriate dimensions in a stable and correct orientation to allow construction of a successful prosthesis. Subsequently the soft tissues surrounding the implant should be able to maintain normal functional integrity and withstand oral hygiene procedures. Aesthetic considerations may be relatively small involving subtle loss of alveolar ridge form or interdental papillae, but at the other extreme may involve significant skeletal jaw base discrepancies which need correction before implant treatment can commence. However, before any corrective surgical procedure is attempted it is important to consider any alternative solutions. For example, potential aesthetic problems may also be overcome by using prosthetic solutions (see Part 9). It is important to discuss the problems and various solutions with the patient, and to explain the relative advantages and disadvantages of these approaches.

Overcoming alveolar bone deficiencies

Implant solutions

As described in Parts 4 and 5, a full assessment of bone height and width (and quality) as well as its relationship to the proposed prosthesis is necessary to allow proper planning for implant surgery. Conventionally the aim is to have a border of 1 mm of bone surrounding the implant at the time of placement. This dictates a minimum bone dimension of 6 mm in both the mesial-distal and bucco-palatal direction to allow an implant of 4 mm diameter to be placed. With narrower ridges the obvious alternative is to use a narrower diameter implant. While there may be merit in considering this option it is important to remember that a reduction in implant size, particularly to a diameter less than 3.5 mm, can greatly reduce implant strength as well as surface area for integration/load distribution. Use of small diameter implants should therefore be restricted to low load situations such as replacement of missing lower incisors or upper lateral incisors. In situations where the ridge is broad but has limited height (less than 10 mm), wider diameter implants up to 6 mm can be used. These have a greater surface area for inte-

gration and load distribution as well as having an increased resistance to fracture. There are now a great many implant configurations to enable placement in regions with little bone volume but long-term data on their success are lacking. Implant placement at an alternative site to facilitate treatment may also be considered, for example using the pterygoid plates or zygomatic buttresses for implant fixation. However, implants placed in these regions may present both surgical and prosthetic difficulties and their use should be limited to experienced clinicians.

Bone augmentation

Deficiencies in bone may be restricted to small, well defined defects involving one or more sites or may be much more generalised in their presentation affecting the entire jaw. Different techniques and materials are therefore employed to augment bone into these areas although a combination may be used to achieve the desired result.

Autogenous bone grafts

Autogenous bone remains the gold standard by which all other materials are judged. It has many advantages over the alternatives in that it is:
- Readily available from adjacent or remote sites
- Sterile
- Biocompatible/non-immunogenic
- Osseoinductive/conductive
- Easy to manipulate.

It may be harvested from intra- and extra-oral sites using trephines or by taking bone blocks or chips. Favoured intra-oral sites include the chin (fig. 1), retromolar areas (fig. 2), and other edentulous areas local or remote to the surgical site. Further bone collection is possible by using surgical bone traps attached to the suction apparatus when taking grafts or preparing implant osteotomy sites. This yields a highly osteoconductive osseous coagulum which is also easy to manipulate. Intra-oral harvesting has many merits in that the surgeon is working in an environment which is familiar, and the graft is of the same developmental origin. However, if there is a requirement for large blocks of bone an alternative site needs to be considered. Larger defects therefore require bone from extra-oral sites, the most common of which is iliac crest. While this donor site can

Autogenous grafts are considered to be the most predictable for replacement of deficient bones to facilitate implant treatment. Augmentation of soft tissue may also be required to improve aesthetics and function.

In this part, we will discuss:
- Overcoming alveolar deficiencies
- Management of localised deficiencies
- Soft tissue deficiencies

[1]Part-time Demonstrator, Guy's and St Thomas' Hospital Trust, London SE1 9RT and Specialist in Periodontics, 21 Wimpole Street, London W1
[2]Professor of Implant Dentistry and Periodontology, Guy's Kings and St Thomas' Medical and Dental School, London SE1 9RT
© British Dental Journal 1999; 187: 532–540

dental implants

provide large blocks of bone, the morbidity associated with this procedure must be considered. Optimisation of grafting is achieved by ensuring that the graft is stable at the time of placement and that there is close adaptation between graft and host bed. This may be achieved by compacting the bone into the available space and by direct fixation using screws or mini-plates (fig. 3). Graft stability may also be improved by using GBR membranes (see below).

In an effort to overcome the morbidity of taking autogenous grafts other techniques and materials have been developed, and these are considered in the following sections.

Guided bone regeneration
One of the most popular techniques used for

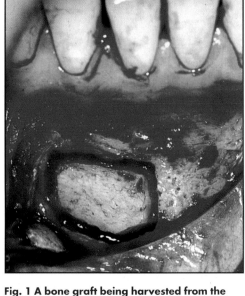

Fig. 1 A bone graft being harvested from the chin. An incision has been made below the mucogingival junction to give access to the bone apical to the incisor teeth. The block graft of cortical and underlying cancellous bone has been outlined with a fissure bur. The lingual cortex is left intact and the block can be elevated from the site

Fig. 3a Corticocancellous block grafts have been firmly fixed to the residual alveolus with self tapping screws. The bone cortex of the recipient site had been perforated with a small round bur to help with revascularisation and union with the graft. Spaces around the bone blocks are then packed with cancellous bone and bone coagulum

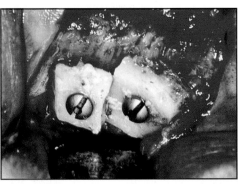

Fig. 3b The grafted area exposed after a period of 4 months. There has been some remodelling but little loss of graft thickness. The retaining screws are removed

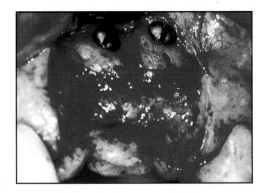

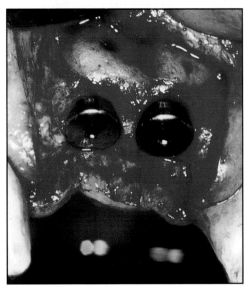

Fig. 3c Two implants have been placed within the grafted area

Fig. 2 Smaller grafts can be harvested from the retromolar area. In this figure two grafts have been taken with a trephine

the treatment of localised ridge deficiencies is guided bone regeneration (GBR). This technique employs barrier membranes which allow creation of a confined defect into which bone progenitor cells may migrate in preference to soft tissue cells, allowing bone to form within the void (fig. 4). Of the many configurations of membranes available one of the most widely used is Gore-Tex™, an expanded polytetrafluoroethylene (PTFE) which was first used in periodontal regeneration. PTFE is non-resorbable and requires removal, therefore involving a second surgical procedure. Other types of membrane are now available which are resorbable and do not require removal.

The ideal properties of GBR membranes are:

- Biocompatible to minimise any inflammatory response. Membranes which incorporate biochemical factors to enhance bone healing are under development
- Occlusive to prevent passage of cells during the healing period. Some membranes are semi permeable and allow passage of fluid whereas others have been tried which are totally impermeable. Totally occlusive materials such as titanium sheets formed into the required shape have also been used
- Physical properties which allow the space under the membrane to be maintained. This may be improved by using: titanium reinforced membranes; 'tent' screws to support the membrane (fig. 5); and fillers such as bone or substitutes to fill the void.
- Enhance wound stability and protection of the initial clot and delicate granulation tissue. Stabilisation of the membrane may be improved by securing it with small screws/pins or the implant cover screw.

In its simplest form GBR can be used to promote bone fill of a defect before implant treatment. It can also be used to regenerate bone in dehiscences and fenestrations around implants at the time of placement (fig. 4), but it must be remembered that any bone thus created does not contribute to initial implant stability and its long-term significance is currently not known.

Wound closure and stability are very important when using GBR and great efforts to maintain the vitality of the overlying soft tissues need to be made. Flaps with wound edges remote from the surgical site are recommended and wound closure without producing any tension in the soft tissues is required. Soft tissue breakdown over sites where membranes are involved can allow bacterial infection, compromised healing and possibly failure of osseointegration.

Alloplastic graft materials

These include materials such as hydroxyapatite, tricalcium phosphate and bioactive glasses. These materials are easy to use and are commonly used as fillers on their own or in combination with autogenous bone. They provide an osteoconductive framework for bone but are not osteoinductive and are unable to contribute to osseointegration. Their use has been widely documented but their efficacy when used alone as grafting materials in implant surgery requires more evaluation with carefully controlled clinical trials, as is the case for many of the bone substitutes.

Hydroxyapatite is available in a variety of forms, from porous resorbable particles to dense non-resorbable and block forms. The commonly used non-resorbable HA becomes embedded in newly formed fibrous tissue and

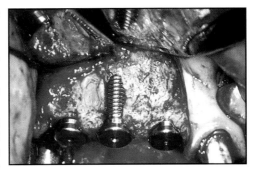

Fig. 4a Maxillary implants placed with a large dehiscence on the middle implant. The small root fragment distal to this was removed and the whole area covered with a Gore-Tex membrane

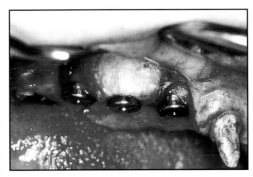

Fig. 4b Surgical exposure of the Gore-Tex membrane after 7 months to remove the membrane and connect healing abutments

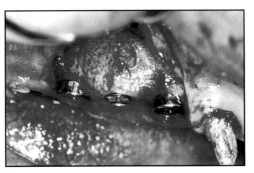

Fig. 4c This shows the bone healing of the area following removal of the membrane. The dehiscence has been covered

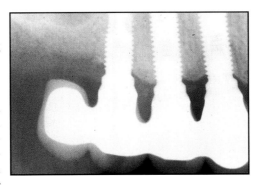

Fig. 4d A radiograph of the same implants following restoration

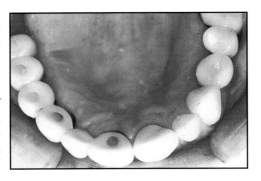

Fig. 4e An occlusal view of the completed restoration showing screw hole access through the fossae and cingulae

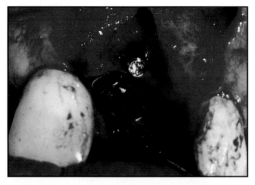

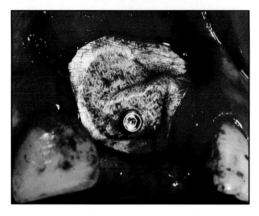

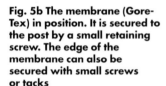

Overcoming alveolar bone deficiencies
- Implant solutions
- Bone augmentation:
  Autogenous bone grafts
  Guided bone
    regeneration
  Alloplastic graft materials
  Allografts
  Xenografts
  Bone promoting
    molecules

bone, and the resulting tissue combination is a less than ideal implant bed.

The new generation of bioactive glasses are an effective synthetic bone grafting material. They are silicate glasses whose main components are sodium, calcium and phosphate in varying combinations in particulate form. They are osteoconductive as well as having bone bonding properties through corrosion of the glass when exposed to bodily fluids to produce a silica gel and a calcium phosphate surface layer. The calcium phosphate layer then recrystallises into hydroxycarbonate apatite which is able to bond to bone. This surface layer bears more similarity to the mineral component of bone than hydroxyapatite.

Allografts
Human bone material in the form of freeze dried bone or demineralised freeze dried bone (DFDB) has been used widely both in periodontology and implant dentistry. The donor bone is harvested from cadavers, processed and sterilised. A wide range of grafts are available, which may be particulate, thin sheets of cortical plate, or much larger bone blocks. They are predominantly used as a scaffold for bone repair and are resorbable but often remain as inert fragments long after placement. Despite the measures taken to ensure sterility and non-infectivity of these grafts some doubt must remain as to their absolute safety.

Xenografts
These are graft materials derived from other animal species. Some have received wide acclaim and are used to provide an inert framework for bone regeneration either alone or in combination with autogenous bone graft. Bio-Oss™ is bovine bone in which the organic component is completely removed to leave the mineralised bone architecture. This renders it non-immunogenic and presumably safe from the possibility of trans-species infection.

Other naturally occurring mineralised substances such as Coral have been advocated as it has a pore size which allows bone ingrowth. Recent research has produced some promising results describing the induction of osteoblasts and mineralised bone following implantation of Nacra (the calcium carbonate shell of molluscs).

Bone promoting molecules
The identification and production of bone morphogenetic proteins are a recent advance in regenerative therapies both in periodontology and implant surgery and hold a lot of promise for the future. They have been used with some success in bone regeneration in the maxillary antrum when delivered in a collagen based sponge. They are also present in their natural form in demineralised freeze dried bone, which may account for the reported efficacy of this material, although the processing may inactivate the bone morphogenetic proteins.

Management of localised deficiencies
Small deficiencies in the alveolar ridge may be treated using simple techniques. It is important to consider whether grafting is necessary to achieve a stable implant at the time of placement or whether it is being used to promote bone repair over exposed areas of the implant. Therefore augmentation of small defects may be considered as preparatory or perioperative procedures.

Before implant placement
Bone augmentation before implant placement is generally the preferred option. This is particularly the case for non-submerged or single stage implants. Alveolar defects should be augmented at least 3 months before implant placement but delays greater than 6 months may result in resorption of the graft.

At implant placement
Implant placement in thin ridges may result in incomplete bone coverage of the implant surface. The resulting defects can be described as either dehiscences involving the marginal bone or more apically located fenestrations (fig. 6). The clinician has to decide whether or not these require bone augmentation using grafts or GBR. This will mainly depend upon the size, location and morphology of the defect. Fenestrations are probably of little clinical significance and usually require no treatment.

However, attempts should be made to repair large dehiscences or the implant placement abandoned and the site grafted to produce a more favourable situation.

Extraction sockets

Most extraction sockets heal perfectly well without interference by the clinician. However, a large defect may be produced if the buccal plate is lost or in cases of long-standing apical or periodontal infection. These defects can be repaired using a variety of techniques including small bone grafts, GBR, or a combination of the two. It is important that any residual infection is eradicated before the implant is placed. Fortunately the removal of the offending tooth and curettage of the socket usually allows this to occur readily.

While it may be possible to improve socket infill at the time of extraction by placing graft material, an alternative is to place an implant immediately into the socket (fig. 7). In this situation the amount of grafting material is significantly reduced by the implant taking up most of the space (fig. 7b). A prerequisite for this technique is that sufficient bone is present to produce initial stability of the implant ie the graft plays no stabilising role at implant place-

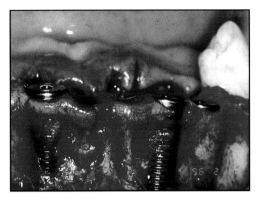

Fig. 6 A large dehiscence with many exposed threads on the implant on the patient's left side. The implant on the patient's right side has a moderate sized fenestration. Augmentation of the bone at the dehiscence site is indicated, whereas the fenestration could be left untreated

ment (fig. 7c). Stability is normally achieved in these situations by engaging sound bone apical to the socket. With the immediate placement technique soft tissue coverage at implant placement can be difficult or impossible to achieve. While this may not be so important for non-submerged implants, it is desirable for submerged systems and cases where grafts, particularly in combination with membranes, are employed. Where soft tissue coverage is considered important the technique of 'delayed immediate placement' may be employed. In such situations the extraction site is left for about 4 to 6 weeks to allow soft tissue healing before an implant is placed. This period can also be useful to allow infections to completely resolve.

Management of larger deficiencies

General techniques

Larger bone deficiencies arise because of long-standing progressive resorption following tooth loss and trauma, developmental anomalies, and pathological conditions (tumour

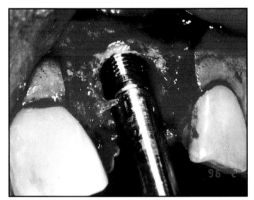

Fig. 7b An implant has been placed in an extraction socket and the residual space is quite small. The implant is firmly anchored in the bone apical to the socket

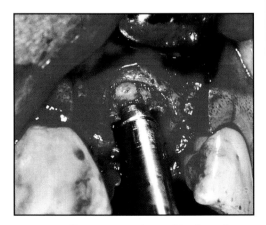

Fig. 7c Small autogenous bone chips have been collected from another intra-oral site and packed into the residual socket

Management of larger deficiencies
• General techniques
• Onlay grafts
• Ridge expansion
• Sinus lifts (sub-antral grafting)
• Inlay grafts combined with maxillary osteotomies
• Bone deficiencies in the posterior mandible

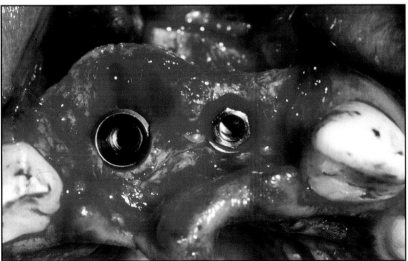

Fig. 7a The two upper central incisors are being replaced with implants. The patient's left incisor was lost many years ago and a standard technique is being employed with placement of a Branemark implant. On the patient's right side the incisor has just been extracted and an implant (Astra) has been placed in the socket. This occupies some of the space within the socket which has good repair potential. Subsequently the labial wall of the socket was collapsed in towards the implant surface thus reducing the bone fill requirement

dental implants

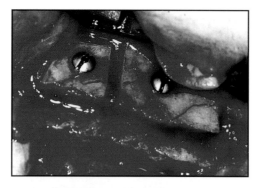

Fig. 8 A thin residual alveolus exists in the posterior maxilla on both sides in this patient. Adequate volumes of autogenous bone could only be obtained from an extra-oral site. In this case iliac crest corticocancellous blocks have been screwed in place to increase the thickness of the ridge. Following a healing period of 3 to 4 months implants can be placed

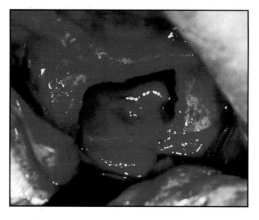

Fig. 9a A window has been carefully cut in the lateral wall of the maxillary sinus. The membrane has been kept intact and the bone window has been pushed inwards, hingeing on the intact membranes. A self contained cavity has thus been created to accept graft material

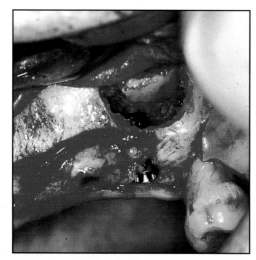

Fig. 9b A smaller sinus elevation. Two implants have been placed within the residual alveolus and protrude into the space created by elevation of the sinus membrane

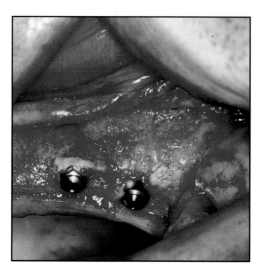

Fig. 9c The cavity has been grafted with autogenous bone harvested from another intra-oral site. This shows a simultaneous sinus elevation, implant placement and graft

resection, cysts, etc). Techniques to overcome these problems, which may involve the entire edentulous jaw, aim to improve the height and or width of the bone available as well as providing bone of sufficient quality to provide implant anchorage. Ridge resorption in the vertical plane may require grafting to allow placement of adequate length implants and to reduce the crown to implant ratio of the prosthesis. Longer implants supporting a lower profile prosthesis will reduce the mechanical demands on the prosthetic components. One of the most difficult problems is the development of a pseudo Class III jaw relation with severe resorption of the edentulous maxilla compared with the mandible. Grafting may therefore be required to provide adequate bone for implant installation and correction of the jaw relationship.

Most of the procedures described in this section are advanced surgical procedures requiring specialist training.

Onlay grafts

Onlay grafts are versatile in that they are able to augment the bone in either the vertical or lateral dimension or a combination of the two (fig. 8). Smaller grafts may be harvested from the chin or retromolar area, although large cortico-cancellous grafts are usually taken from the iliac crest. Grafts should be secured to the recipient bed using miniscrews and plates or wires. The host bed is perforated with a small bur to allow blood clot to form between the two bone surfaces and to allow communication with the cancellous bone which contains osteoprogenitor cells. Any remaining voids may be packed with cancellous bone chips to maximise the healing potential.

A modification of this technique has been described where implants are used to stabilise large onlay grafts. In these cases an iliac graft is taken in one piece which is the same dimension as the proposed dental arch by using a surgical template. The graft is secured to the residual ridge using six or more implants. This is a useful technique to alter jaw relations and simultaneously place implants but requires that the residual alveolus is capable of stabilising the implants and graft.

Ridge expansion

Lack of bone in the bucco-lingual direction may also be dealt with by mid-crestal expansion in which a central cleft is created with standard osteotomes and the ridge split longitudinally. It is important to limit the spread of the longitudinal split by using transverse cuts through the alveolus at both ends of the ridge. Once expanded to the desired width the void can be grafted or a combination of implants and graft material may be placed. As a one stage technique problems may arise because of poor initial stability of the implant. Case selection using this technique is critical as brittle bone may fracture in an unpredictable fashion causing further bone loss. Further accurate positioning and orientation of the implants may be difficult to achieve.

Sinus lifts (sub-antral grafting)

The sinus lift or sinus floor elevation is similar to a Caldwell-Luc procedure combined with grafting of the floor of the maxillary sinus (fig. 9). It is a procedure that can be performed under local anaesthesia and involves carefully cutting a window in the lateral antral wall using surgical burs but retaining the integrity of the sinus membrane (fig. 9b). The window may then be in-fractured to create a discrete cavity on the superior aspect of the residual alveolus. Graft material may then be inserted which serves to keep the bone 'trap-door' in its elevated position (fig. 9c). If the sinus membrane is torn it is not advisable to graft particulate material although blocks of corticocancellous bone can be secured in position. The technique is commonly used as a pre-implant procedure when the residual alveolar ridge has resorbed to a point where initial implant stability is compromised. Thus maxillary ridges with less than 5 mm of available bone height should be augmented at least 3 months before implant placement. This protocol increases the likelihood of achieving stable implants at placement and improves the overall success rates. Alternatively sinus lifts may be employed to allow installation of a longer implant without it entering the sinus proper. If performed as a one stage procedure the implant serves as a support for the bone 'trap door' and may also be used to fix the graft in place, particularly if a block of cortico-cancellous bone is used.

Inlay grafts combined with maxillary osteotomies

Gross resorption of the maxilla leading to a Class III skeletal relationship can be treated using an inlay graft combined with a Le Fort I type osteotomy. This will improve the skeletal jaw relationship and available bone height while leaving the alveolar crest form unchanged. This is therefore particularly useful in the pseudo Class III edentulous maxilla or in partially dentate individuals requiring orthognathic surgery. Once the Le Fort I down fracture is complete a bone inlay of predetermined thickness is placed in the void and sandwiched between the two sections and secured using mini-plates. The size of the inlay required necessitates the use of cortico-cancellous bone from the iliac crest for this procedure.

Bone deficiencies in the posterior mandible

Alveolar resorption in the posterior part of the mandible eventually reduces the available bone height above the inferior dental canal to a point where implants cannot be placed without risk of injury to the inferior dental bundle. It is important to emphasise that due consideration has to be given when planning not only for the implant length but for the fact that the drills used usually prepare the osteotomy site 1–2 mm deeper than the actual implant. It is therefore imperative that the surgeon is familiar with the system and drills being used when planning surgery close to important anatomical structures.

Lack of height above the ID canal can be overcome by onlay grafts or alternatively the nerve bundle itself may be surgically transposed. This is a difficult technique involving deroofing the nerve and dissecting the neurovascular bundle from the body of the mandible as far distally as is required. Implants may then be placed spanning the entire height of the mandible while avoiding the nerve. Once the implants are in place, the boney window which was removed from over the nerve may be replaced in a more mesial position with the nerve emerging from the more distal aspect. This technique carries a potentially high morbidity and should be used rarely and by experienced surgeons. In the edentulous mandible it may be preferable to place multiple fixtures anterior to the mental foramen and construct a prosthesis with a distal cantilever.

Soft tissue deficiencies

Soft tissue deficiencies can give rise to both functional and aesthetic problems.

Functional problems

The soft tissue cuff around the implant abutment has to withstand oral hygiene practices and shearing forces during mastication. It is therefore desirable (but not essential) to have the implant emerging through keratinised attached mucosa. Proposed implant sites that are deficient in this tissue may be augmented by using free gingival grafts either before implant placement, at the time of implant placement, or at abutment connection. Free gingival grafts can be taken from the palate and placed on a prepared donor site which has a good vascular supply (fig. 10). As an alternative interpositional connective tissue grafts may be placed to augment the soft tissue.

Aesthetic problems

Small defects in gingival contour may improve once the restoration emerges through the gingiva. The contours of the restorative components may provide enough support to the soft tissue to give them a perfectly satisfactory appearance without the need for grafting (figs 11 and 12). In addition remodelling of the soft tissues can continue for some time after the prosthesis has been placed.

However, larger more obvious soft tissue

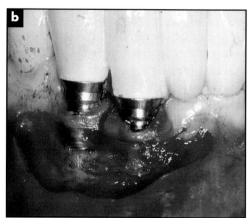

Fig. 10 a) There is complete lack of keratinised attached tissue on the buccal aspect of these two implants. The patient had experienced considerable discomfort and a free gingival graft was advised. b) A graft bed is prepared by making a split thickness dissection. c) A graft taken from the palate is transferred and sutured in position. This free graft initially receives nutrients from plasma exuding from the graft bed. Rapid vascularisation then occurs.
d) The healed graft after 10 days. This will provide a zone of tissue which will be easier for the patient to maintain in health

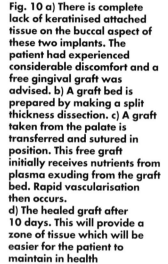

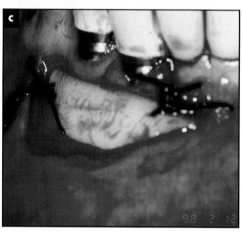

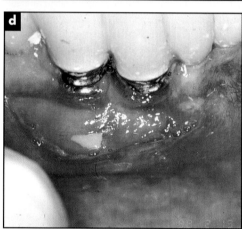

Fig. 11 a) An edentulous space in the upper canine region. An implant was placed 6 months previously and abutment connection surgery is to be carried out. The profile of the ridge is very flat. b) The implant was exposed, an abutment connected, and a provisional crown (with a good emergence profile) constructed and fitted. The profile of the soft tissue has been considerably enhanced

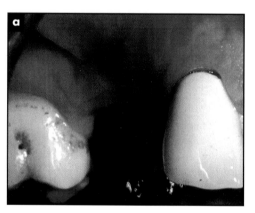

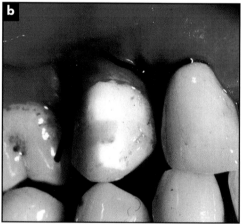

Fig. 12 a) A patient requiring replacement of an upper central incisor. There is a marked ridge deformity but the patient did not want to undergo grafting procedures. b) The completed single tooth implant. There is no aesthetic deformity because the emergence of the crown through the soft tissue has eliminated it

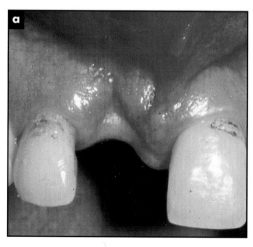

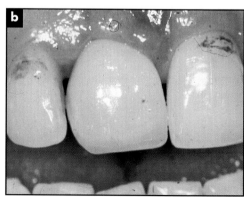

defects will require grafting and this is best performed as a preparatory procedure before implant placement. It can also be performed at the time of implant placement but it may be extremely difficult (or impossible) after the prosthesis has been fitted.

The ideal augmentation material is the patient's own tissue and both free gingival and connective tissue grafts can usually be used to deal with all but the most severe soft tissue deficiencies. Larger deficiencies will also require augmentation of the hard tissues.

Interdental papillary regeneration has been the cause of much surgical enterprise during the past few years and is desirable particularly in the partially dentate patient and around single tooth implants. The papillary regeneration technique basically involves preservation and rotation of attached gingiva at the time of abutment connection surgery. While this is undoubtedly a valid technique, natural papillary remodelling occurs around single teeth and limited span bridges once the prosthesis has been in place for some time. This stands as testimony to the ultimate biocompatability of the well made implant reconstruction and the soft tissue moulding effect of a prosthesis with anatomical emergence profiles.

Conclusion

It can be seen therefore that a myriad of solutions exist to overcome anatomical problems. It is important however to remember the desired treatment outcome and to explore all the possible solutions. By keeping the techniques as simple and predictable as possible and using the patients own tissue the likelihood of success increases greatly.

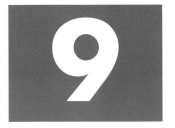

Advanced restorative techniques

Leslie Howe,[1] Paul Palmer,[2] and Vincent Barrett,[3]

Great importance has already been placed on the need for very careful planning prior to embarking on implant treatment in order to try and obtain the best possible outcome. Unfortunately there are situations where a less than ideal implant position has been achieved either by design, perhaps to overcome an anatomic problem, or because of an error at the surgical stage. It is easy to blame the surgical stage for later prosthodontic problems but in the real world, even with surgeons who have a lot of experience, there are many factors which can effect the final position of the implant which cannot be identified until the time of operation. If surgeon and prosthodontist are working as a team it is essential that the surgeon has been provided with as much information as possible, such as stents, and is aware of 'second choice' implant sites if the prime site proves to be unusable. The worst possible scenario is for

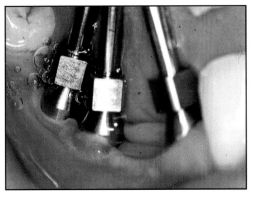

Fig. 2 Impression copings magnify any convergence of implants. Care must be taken to alter copings so that they do not touch

the implant to be placed in the easiest bony site without regard to the final restoration. Even movement of the implant by 1–2 mm can have a dramatic effect on outcome with restorations at the front of the mouth (fig. 1).

Patients may feel that an implant will restore them to their original appearance. They must therefore be informed that because of soft and hard tissue loss there may be an element of compromise involved.

If implants are placed in a difficult position to restore there are a multitude of alternative prosthodontic solutions available.

What are the potential problems?
Most problems can be overcome with strict attention to the guidelines given in Parts 3 and 4, such as the use of diagnostic dentures and wax-ups followed by surgical stents. Most importantly, patient expectations should be realistic with an accurate representation of them prior to treatment of what can be achieved and what the end result is likely to be.

Implant positioning
Errors in mesio-distal spacing may result in implants which are too close or distant to adjacent teeth or implants. If implants are too close it may be difficult to contour the restoration to allow for adequate oral hygiene or produce an aesthetic tooth shape. It can also be difficult to fit abutment components and take impressions as there are minimum dimensions for components (fig. 2).

Alternatively, widely spaced implants may require oversized crowns or placing narrow

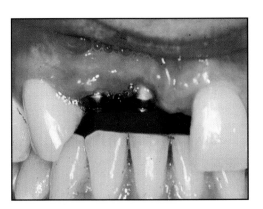

Fig. 1a Implants placed in the upper right incisor sites with healing abutments visible. Because of a large incisive canal the central incisor implant is placed too distally

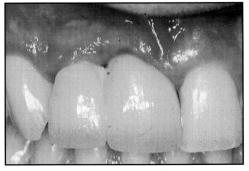

Fig. 1b Crowns in place revealing an irregular gingival margin to the central incisor. The resulting interdental space will be difficult to clean

> **Many alternative techniques are available to ensure the best possible outcome for an implant restoration.**

In this part, we will discuss:
- What are the potential problems?
- Special techniques
- Particular problem areas

[1]Consultant in Restorative Dentistry, Guy's and St Thomas' Hospitals Trust, London SE1 9RT and Specialist in Restorative Dentistry and Prosthodontics, 21 Wimpole Street, London W1M 7AD; [2]Part-time Demonstrator, Guy's, Kings and St Thomas' Medical and Dental School, London SE1 9RT and Specialist in Periodontics, 21 Wimpole Street, London W1M 7AD; [3]Private Practitioner, 38 Devonshire Street, London W1

dental implants

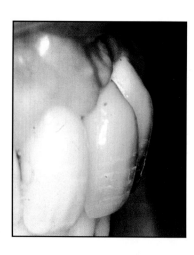

Fig. 3 Implant supported crowns have to mimic the natural curvature of the adjacent natural teeth. In this case the gingival margin of the implant crowns is high because of alveolar resorption

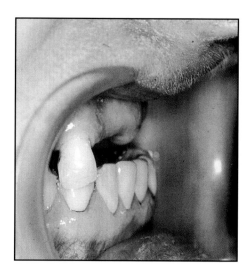

Fig. 4 Resorption of the upper ridge will make it difficult for a fixed implant supported bridge to have an anterior Class 1 incisor relationship. A removable implant supported overdenture should be considered

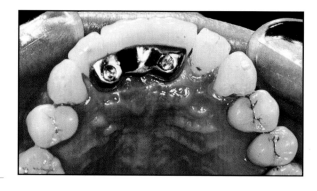

Fig. 5 Angled abutments have produced a bulky palatal contour

What are the potential problems?
- Implant positioning
- Patient expectations and appearance
- Function and speech
- Presence of existing teeth

double pontics which may look unaesthetic. It should be remembered that different implant and abutment diameters can be selected and the particular width of the tooth to be replaced should be compatible.

Problems may result from the angulation of the implant, either in relation to other implants or to the desired position of the final restoration. This may occur because the shape of the remaining alveolar ridge has dictated the implant angulation or perhaps the patients' natural teeth have a curved contour, in particular a marked angle between crown and root (fig. 3).

The vertical space between the implant head and the opposing dentition may be limited and

conventional components may not fit. In addition the interalveolar relationships may create a discrepancy between implant position and desired tooth placement. For example, the Class 2 div 2 incisor relationship may call for the use of angled components or where significant alveolar resorption has occurred on one arch but natural teeth remain in the opposing jaw (fig. 4).

Patient expectations and appearance
Patients who have worn dentures with a labial flange are used to the appearance of a restored gingival and alveolar contour, and may be disappointed if this does not exist in their new restoration.

Implant treatment is complex, lengthy and expensive, and patients often become more demanding with time during their treatment and significantly more critical than they would have been with a simpler restoration provided in less time. Beware the patient who says at the start that the appearance is not important. When restoring a tooth in the upper anterior region many patients will demand a good result, not just of the tooth shade but also of the whole tooth/gingival complex, such as the gingival margin and the interdental papilla.

Function and speech
It is rare for implant supported restorations not to provide for good function even in a difficult restorative situation, however sometimes the treatment will focus problems onto existing teeth or previous restorations which may have been satisfactory before. In contrast speech can often be affected with upper anterior restorations. This is normally transitory but may be persistent if bulky components are used which overcontour the palatal surface (fig. 5).

Excessively large embrasure spaces combined with a loss of interdental papillae may result in air and saliva being expressed which upsets some patients. This may be rectified by using spoilers or removable acrylic veneers.

Presence of existing teeth
In general, it is recommended that implants should not be joined to natural teeth with a fixed restoration. However, it may be necessary or desirable to include natural teeth into an implant reconstruction, perhaps because insufficient implants could be placed and the extra support of a sound tooth could help (fig. 6). In some cases a sound tooth occupies space between edentulous areas and can be incorporated into the new restoration, although some clinicians would prefer to extract the tooth.

Retaining teeth can help aesthetics by preserving alveolar form. Teeth can be incorporated into a restoration using gold copings or precision attachments, however the degree of support provided by teeth in such a restoration is debatable. As the implants are essentially ankylosed it is likely that the teeth contribute little support which sometimes shows as infra-eruption.

Special techniques

Traditional restorative techniques for implant restorations involve choosing the abutment, placing it and then taking an impression. A gold framework can then be manufactured and the final aesthetic surface applied. This approach is fine if the case is straightforward and the implants are in the ideal place. If however there is a problem, identifying this too late can result in having to change abutments or repeating laboratory work which can be expensive and time consuming. Special techniques are therefore available to overcome this.

Implant position impressions (head of fixture impressions)

Rather than take impressions at the abutment level, most manufacturers produce impression copings that record the exact position of the implant in relation to adjacent teeth and soft tissues. Impression copings are attached to the implant using guide pins and a 'pick up' technique is employed (fig. 7).

Following attachment of an implant analogue, a model can be produced which, with a soft tissue mask, will allow the operator and technician to choose the ideal abutment and technique for the case (fig. 8).

For single teeth and short span bridges this working cast is considered accurate enough to proceed with construction of the restoration using the actual abutment screwed onto the model. With longer span bridges it may be desirable to replace the abutments in the mouth and retake further impressions in the conventional way.

Diagnostic frameworks

Following impression taking, rather than proceeding with the definitive framework which may dictate tooth position early on, it is often desirable to have a full diagnostic try-in using acrylic and wax. The simplest approach is to construct an acrylic partial denture based on the implant position. More accurately, the bridge cylinders can be linked together with acrylic or light cured composite and the tooth contours waxed on top, or denture teeth placed in wax to reproduce the possible end result (fig. 9). This also allows the clinician to check the accuracy of the cast. Any problems with fit can be rectified by sectioning the try-in and rejoining.

The trial restoration can then be tried in the mouth for the patient to see and any adjustments carried out. The agreed result can be returned to the laboratory and a putty mask

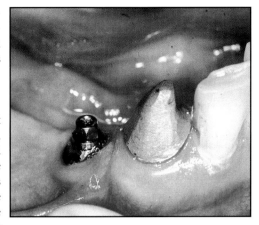

Fig. 6a Only one implant could be placed distal to the canine tooth because of resorption and the inferior dental canal. To provide the patient with two premolar teeth the implant is linked to the adjacent tooth. A gold coping is used to protect the tooth if decementation should occur

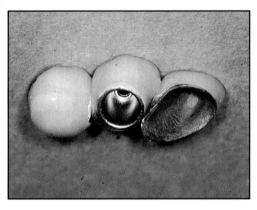

Fig. 6b The completed bridge showing a distally cantilevered pontic

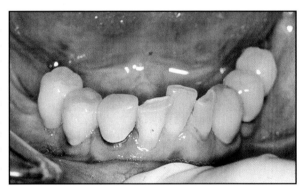

Fig. 6c The bridge in place. There is also a conventional implant supported bridge on the other side of the jaw

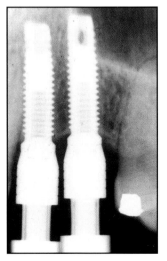

Fig. 7a Radiograph of the head of implant impression copings in place to verify seating

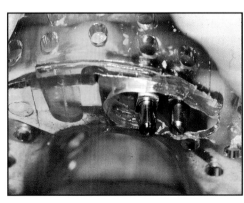

Fig. 7b The retaining pins project through a window in a stock tray for a 'pick up' impression

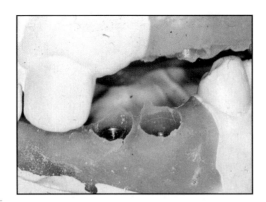

Fig. 8a Impression of implant heads with a soft tissue mask on the cast

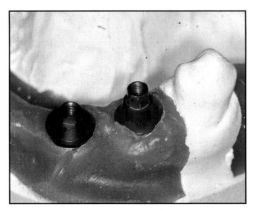

Fig. 8b Analogues of suitable abutments can be tried in to ensure the correct choice is made

taken to ensure the definitive restoration copies it. The framework can be made to properly support the tooth position by cutting back from the wax teeth.

Several manufacturers now produce temporary cylinders that can be used for provisional or diagnostic restorations. These directly screw onto the implant without the need for a conventional abutment and allow even more flexibility in the decision taking until all of the potential problems have been identified. They are particularly useful in complex transitional cases.

Screwed or cemented restorations

Traditional techniques were developed to construct short or long span bridges using pre-made components that were cast together and held in place with gold screws. Conventional cemented techniques were used only in single tooth implant restorations. Although the significant advantage of easy retrievability and an excellent marginal fit of pre-made screwed components is very attractive, many operators have found the complex laboratory processes involved outweigh the advantages (Table 1). Several techniques for cemented restorations are now popular.

In the same way that conventional abutments can be chosen, prepable abutments can be chosen for height, width and angulation. These can be placed on an implant position model and trimmed to mimic tooth preparations. A conventional bridge can then be made and cemented. Of particular advantage is the ability to choose abutments that correspond to the width and contour of the tooth to be replaced (fig. 10).

Although abutment preparations can be carried out in the mouth, normally only final finishing is recommended and the bulk of the work is carried out in the laboratory.

Cemented restorations

As already described, prepable abutments which allow conventional crown and bridgework can be supplied by most manufacturers and are chosen so that the gingival margin for the final restoration can be placed just subgingivally in the labial and proximal areas. A natural emergence angle can be developed and the soft tissue modified with a provisional restoration. Ideally this can be developed at the abutment connection stage by taking a

Table 1	Advantages and disadvantages of screw retained versus cemented restorations	
	Advantages	**Disadvantages**
Screw	Easily retrievable	Accurate framework required for passive fit
	Machined accurate components	Implant position/angulation critical
	Screw acts as fail safe component	Potential for screw fracture and loosening
		Screw-hole may spoil the appearance
Cemented	Customised abutment is highly flexible	Difficult to retrieve
	Can join teeth and implants more readily	Harder laboratory technique
		Temporary bridge normally required
	Small discrepancies in fit are filled by cement lute	Conventional impression can lead to errors in fit
	Comparable with 'ordinary dentistry'	Potential for excess cement
		May encourage a lower standard of clinical and technical acceptability

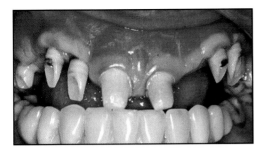

Fig. 9a Plastic abutment analogues are tried in for this complex case

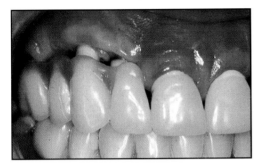

Fig. 9b A diagnostic wax-up of the desired tooth position in relation to the abutments can then be tried in prior to any metal castings

simple impression at first stage surgery and constructing a temporary restoration while the implant is integrating to be fitted at second stage surgery. This allows the soft tissue to heal around a more ideal contour. It also provides the patient with a good temporary restoration without the need to modify pre-existing temporary restorations to fit around healing abutments.

Some manufacturers produce prepable abutments to allow an in-built angulation between implant and restoration. There is some scope for adjustment of the angulation with standard prepable abutments but this is limited by the need to retain bulk around the screwhole for the abutment screw. Alternatively, fully customised abutments can be made using conventional waxing and casting techniques with burn-out or precious metal templates to fit the implant head (fig. 11).

Much has been written in the literature about the need for a passive fit for any casting that is screw retained. It would seem that this is an ideal that is rarely attained and its importance has possibly been over emphasised. Introducing a cement lute allows for small discrepancies in fit to be insignificant. Normally the final restoration is only cemented with a weak cement which allows the possibility for removal if necessary. Small lateral grub screws or a single conventional screwed abutment can be incorporated into the design to give the patient security that the bridge will not be suddenly displaced. Fortunately, decementation of implant restorations does not result in caries! Natural teeth incorporated into any cemented structure should ideally have a permanently cemented

gold coping under the bridge structure so that subsequent bridge removal or debonding will not result in damage to the tooth.

Screw retained restorations
Many clinicians still prefer the simplicity and retrievability of screw retention and patients who have experienced the problems of failing conventional bridge work often appreciate the advantages. Implant positioning is however critical if the screw access hole is to be non-visible and in the ideal site.

On occasions it may be necessary to correct the position of the screw hole by selecting an angled abutment (which are available in a variety of angles). Selection is made easier using a head of implant impression and analogues tried in the laboratory. The final restoration is either based on standard abutment gold cylinders or customised superstructures. Ideally, with any screw retained restoration, fully machined and prefabricated components are preferred to ensure an accurate fit under screw tightening. With angled abutments aesthetics can be a problem unless the implant has been placed quite deeply as the abutment collar can show on the labial aspect.

Angled abutments can also create phonetic

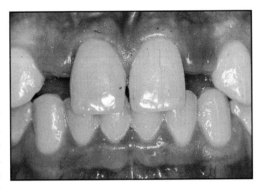

Fig. 10a Missing upper lateral incisors where the width of the spaces is only 5 mm

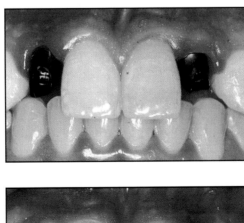

Fig. 10b Narrow width prepable abutments can be produced

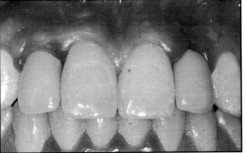

Fig. 10c Crowns immediately after cementation

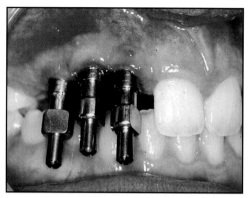

Fig. 11a Surgical placement of these implants in the thin ridge has resulted in a labial angulation. With a screw retained bridge the access holes for the screws would be visible. A customised cemented bridge is therefore indicated

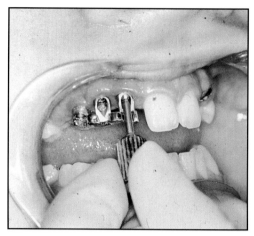

Fig. 11b A jig is used to locate the abutments to one another to ensure their correct relationship

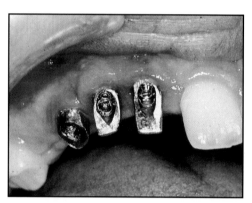

Fig. 11c Customised cast gold abutments in place

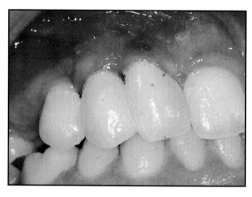

Fig. 11d Completed bridge

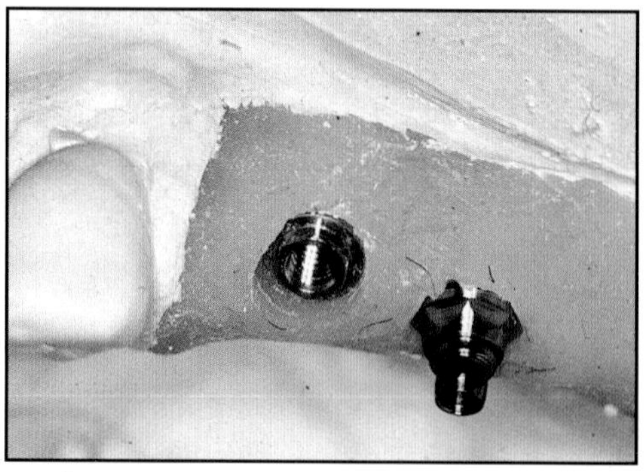

Fig. 12a The head of implant impression shows that the mesial implant is quite superficial and any metal abutment would show. The distal abutment is in a conventional position

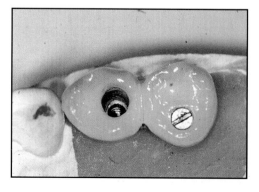

Fig. 12b A bridge is constructed combining the abutment into the bridge to allow the porcelain to be extended down to the implant head. The result is a larger access hole on the occlusal surface for the abutment screw

and oral hygiene difficulties because of the increased bulk of abutment. Difficulties can arise in correctly placing the abutments into the mouth as they need to seat in the desired position on the anti-rotational element of the implant. A locating jig can be made to facilitate this (fig. 11b).

Although abutments are available in a variety of collar heights, problems can arise when there is minimal occlusal height available, for example, under 7 mm for a Branemark implant, as there is little room to place an aesthetic plug into the access hole to cover the screw. Shorter abutments (minimum profile abutments) are available which allow restorations with a 5 mm occlusal space.

Superficially placed implants where there is little occlusal space and where the collar of the head of the implant is near the surface can present major aesthetic problems if the metal collar of the abutment is visible. Abutments are available for the Branemark implant to allow the abutment and restoration to be incorporated into one unit, the UCLA abutment. This allows the restoration (porcelain) margin to extend down to the head of the implant. The disadvantage of this approach is the need for a larger screw access hole to allow for the abutment screw (fig. 12).

Replacing missing soft tissue

Soft and hard tissue grafting techniques are often the preferred way of dealing with this problem particularly in isolated defects. However, many patients are not keen to undergo further surgery and prefer to accept some level of compromise in the final appearance. The days of the traditional Branemark implant supported 'oil rig' restoration approach, particularly in the upper jaw, is no longer acceptable for most patients although the ease of maintenance of these cases is obvious. Extension of pink acrylic or porcelain can help (fig. 13), but care must be taken to ensure cleansibility. Extensions or fixed flanges (spoilers) projecting in front of abutments is a tempting solution particularly if the implant is in a poor position, but usually makes access for oral hygiene impossible. Removable flanges may not be well tolerated by patients and are difficult to maintain.

In a situation where significant amounts of tissue are missing leading to aesthetic and phonetic difficulties and the patient will not accept an implant stabilised over-denture, then a milled bar linking the implants with a (patient) removable bridge superstructure retained by locking pins can be considered. This is an elegant but complex approach with significant cost implications.

Particular problem areas

Single teeth restorations

The deeper the implant is sited the easier it is to overcome angulation and position problems and develop an ideal emergence profile. When interdental papillae are absent the crown may need to be slightly overcontoured proximally to help support and encourage development of soft tissue and close dark triangular spaces (fig. 15).

If the soft tissue overlying the abutment area is thin and a metal abutment might cause greying of the gingiva, an all porcelain abutment can be used. This is a relatively new development and long-term data are not available but initial results are very promising (fig. 16).

Short spans

The major problem with short spans is the temptation to put implants too close together leading to crowns with a poor appearance. Sometimes, if too many implants have been placed too close together, the decision has to be taken to not use one of the implants and construct a bridge using the remainder (fig. 17).

Full arch bridges

In many ways these restorations, particularly in the lower jaw where appearance is not paramount, are proving to be the easiest to provide. In the upper jaw it is often best to avoid placing

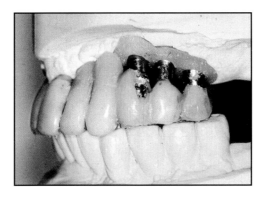

Fig. 13a A 10-year-old 'oil rig' style bridge has been removed from the mouth with its conventional abutments and is seated on a new model

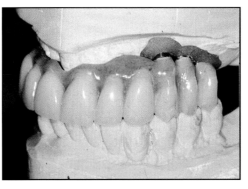

Fig. 13b With shorter bridge abutments and extended acrylic work the visible metal can be eliminated

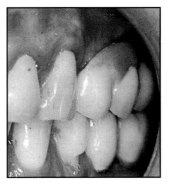

Fig. 14a A spoiler was used to disguise visible metal abutments

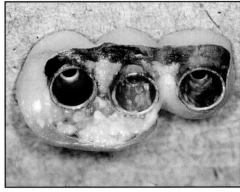

Fig. 14b Such a fixed restoration was impossible for the patient to clean

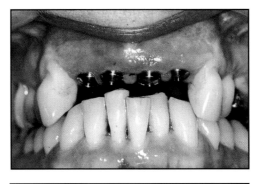

Fig. 15a Four missing upper incisor teeth with a resulting flat ridge. The healing abutments are in place

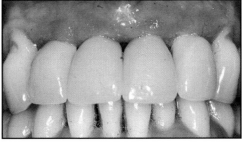

Fig 15b To reduce the dark triangular spaces that would result from the lack of papillae the final crowns are overcontoured cervically

dental implants

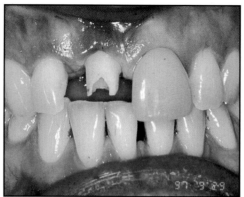

Fig 16a All porcelain abutment in place

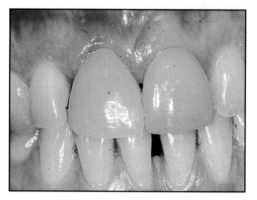

Fig 16b All porcelain crown cemented with a tooth coloured cement

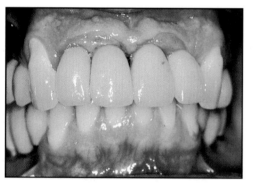

Fig 17a Four anterior crowns placed in a resorbed ridge that is now too narrow from canine to canine

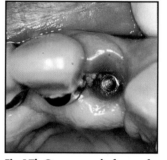

Fig 17b On removal of one of the crowns, the difficulty in cleaning can be easily seen. Note the absence of healthy interdental tissue

implants in the incisor sites so that the operator/ technician can place these teeth in the ideal position, not dictated by the implant position, to achieve ideal aesthetics. If the bone volume is adequate the canine and premolar sites are therefore to be preferred.

The difficulties of achieving a good fit for screw retention has led many to prefer the cemented approach for these long spans. It should be remembered that if multiple implants of sufficient length have been placed a potential long span bridge can often be split up into multiple smaller units.

Conclusion

The prefabricated components available can make the prosthodontic treatment of patients with ideally positioned implants a straight-forward procedure. However, when any degree of variation from the ideal is encountered the prosthodontist can have a difficult time satisfying the patients' expectations. Implant systems should therefore be chosen with a broad range of prosthodontic components available.

In summary, start with a clear idea of the desired result and try this in the patient's mouth. By taking an impression of the implant position and relating this to the desired end result, suitable abutments can be chosen. In any complex situation it is advisable to proceed to a full try in before the superstructure is made to ensure that the abutment choice and aesthetics are correct. Above all, the surgeon should work with the prosthodontic end point in mind, to minimise the risk of an unsatisfactory aesthetic or functional restoration.

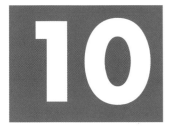

Complications and maintenance

Richard Palmer,[1] Paul Palmer,[2] and Leslie Howe,[3]

The proposed success criteria for dental implant systems were described in Part 1. It has been suggested that longitudinal studies of implant systems should be a minimum of 5 years (preferably prospective studies rather than retrospective), with adequate radiographic and clinical supporting data to determine the level of failure and complication rate. As described in previous chapters, failure of osseointegration of individual implants should be relatively rare, with most failures occurring during the initial healing period or following abutment connection and initial loading. Longer term complications are associated with general wear and tear, inadequate attention to oral hygiene, poorly controlled occlusal forces, poor design of prostheses or use of an inadequately tested implant system.

Maintenance requirements and complications vary widely between patients, depending on susceptibility to caries and periodontal disease in the dentate patients, complexity and type of implant supported prostheses, functional demands and the patient's ability to attain an adequate standard of oral hygiene.

Re-evaluation of the implant retained prosthesis

It is generally recommended that patients treated with implant prostheses are seen at least on an annual basis, but in many cases they will also require routine hygienist treatment at 3, 4 or 6 monthly intervals according to individual requirements. At each re-evaluation appointment the following should be reviewed:

Condition of the prosthesis/restoration

The prostheses should be checked for signs of wear or breakage. Fixed restorations should have the cementation or screw fixation checked. This may include checking the screws which retain the prostheses and those which retain the abutments (see below). The occlusion should be re-evaluated, particularly where there has been occlusal wear of the prostheses or co-existing natural dentition. In published longitudinal studies of implant systems it was necessary to remove fixed bridge superstructures to evaluate the success of individual implants. However, this is not generally recommended in normal patient follow-up unless there is suspicion that there is a problem with one of the implants. Fixed prostheses which

have proved difficult to clean by the patient may require removal to allow adequate professional cleaning, which is easier with screw retained fixed prostheses than cemented types.

Removable prostheses need to be checked for retention and stability. In the case of prostheses with combined implant and mucosal support it is important to check that the implants are not suffering from overload caused by loss of mucosal support because of further ridge resorption. It has been suggested that removable prostheses often require more maintenance in the form of adjustment and replacement of retentive elements such as clips and 'ball retainers', compared with fixed prostheses.

Screw retention and crown cementation

Multiple units are more likely to be screw retained whereas the majority of single units are cemented. The screws retaining a prosthesis to the abutment are often covered with a layer of restorative material, such as composite or glass ionomer, which may need replacing. Screws which are accessible should be checked to ensure that they have not loosened. This is more likely to occur in an ill-fitting prostheses or where high loads have been applied (see the section on Implant Component Failure).

Crown decementation of single tooth units is unusual, even in cases where a relatively weak temporary cement has been used. This is because of the close fit of the abutment to the crown, and in some cases a high degree of parallelism between them which may make separation impossible. A more common complication is failure to seat the crown at the original cementation because of failure to relieve hydraulic pressure within the crown using a cementation vent (fig. 1). The resulting poor marginal fit and exposure of a large amount of cement lute may result in soft tissue inflammation because of the increased bacterial plaque retention. A vent also helps to reduce excess cement being extruded at the crown margins which can give rise to considerable inflammation, including soft tissue abscess and fistula formation. Plaque retention and development of inflammation may also be the initial sign of a loose abutment (see below).

Abutment connection

Repeated chewing cycles may produce abutment loosening and development of a gap

> **Maintenance requirements vary with the complexity of treatment provided. In well planned and treated cases, complications should be rare.**

> **In this part, we will discuss:**
> - Re-evaluation of the implant retained prosthesis
> - Routine hygiene treatment requirements
> - Management of other specific complications

[1]Professor of Implant Dentistry and Periodontology, Guy's Kings and St Thomas' Medical and Dental School, London SE1 9RT [2]Part-time Demonstrator, Guy's and St Thomas' Hospital Trust, London SE1 9RT and Specialist in Periodontics, 21 Wimpole Street, London W1 [3]Consultant in Restorative Dentistry, Guy's and St Thomas' Hospitals Trust, London SE1 9RT and Specialist in Restorative Dentistry and Prosthodontics, 21 Wimpole Street, London W1M 7AD

dental implants

Fig. 1 A radiograph of a single tooth implant replacing an upper canine. There is a large gap between the crown and the abutment because of failure to seat the crown properly during cementation. The fact that the crown did not interfere with the occlusion suggests that the original fault was failure to seat the impression coping — the crown was therefore made to fit an abutment at the wrong level

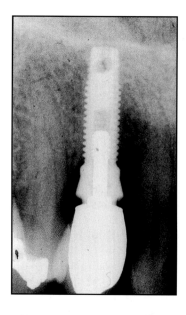

Fig. 2 There is considerable inflammation in the labial soft tissues surrounding this single tooth implant replacing the upper left central incisor. The patient had suffered a severe blow to the crown which had bent and loosened the abutment screw. The resultant subgingival gap had allowed bacterial infection. The situation was corrected with replacement and tightening of the abutment screw

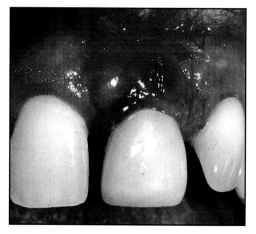

between abutment and implant. This complication can be largely prevented by attention to occlusal contacts and adequate tightening of the abutment screw in the first place by using specifically designed torque wrenches/hand pieces. Variations in the designs of abutment/implant interface such as the morse taper of the ITI system, or internal conical seal of the Astra system, should reduce the occurrence of this complication. Abutment loosening is more likely to occur in patients with a parafunctional activity, in situations where inadequate attention has been paid to the occlusal contacts in all excursions, and rarely when the crown has been subjected to accidental trauma (fig. 2). Most single tooth restorations have cemented crowns with no direct access to the abutment for screw tightening. Therefore, should this be required, removal of the crown is necessary. It is important to note that under circumstances of direct trauma it is preferable to have a design system where hopefully a weaker and more easily replaceable component is damaged.

Status of the soft tissue

The standard of oral hygiene should be evaluated and the presence of supragingival calculus noted

(see later the section on Routine Hygiene Treatment Requirements). The mucosa surrounding the implant abutments at the emerging restorations should appear free of superficial inflammation. The transmucosal part of the implant restoration may emerge through non-keratinised mucosa, particularly in situations where there has been severe loss of bone eg edentulous jaws. In contrast, many restorations emerge through soft tissue which appears very similar to adjacent keratinised gingiva. There are considerable differences between the appearances of these tissues, in that the non-keratinised mucosa will appear red, possibly more mobile and will have visible blood vessels within it. Gentle pressure on the exterior surface of the soft tissue should not result in any bleeding or exudate and will produce minimal discomfort. Probing depths may be evaluated but will depend upon the thickness of the original mucosa (see Part 2) and any overgrowth of gingival tissue which may have occurred. Ideally probing depths should be relatively shallow (< 4 mm) with no bleeding. If increased probing depths, soft tissue proliferation, copious bleeding, exudate or tenderness to pressure are found (fig. 3), the area should be examined radiographically (regardless of whether radiographic re-evaluation is scheduled) to determine whether there has been any loss of marginal bone or loss of integration. In these circumstances it may be advisable to dismantle the implant superstructure to allow adequate examination of individual abutments and implants.

Radiographic evaluation

Radiographs (fig. 4) are frequently used in implant treatment to evaluate:

- Initial osseointegration
- Seating of abutments
- Fit of prostheses
- Baseline bone level evaluation following completion of prosthetic treatment
- Longitudinal evaluation of bone levels.

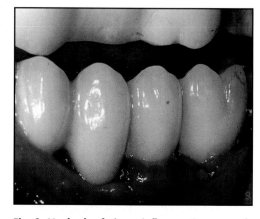

Fig. 3. Marked soft tissue inflammation around a mandibular bridge. The embrasure spaces were tight and the patient found it difficult to clean

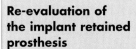

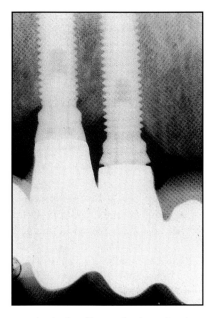

Fig. 4 A periapical radiograph of two implants incorporated in a fixed bridge showing a number of important features. In both implants the thread profiles are clearly visible confirming good paralleling technique. The implant on the left side has the bone crest coincident with the top thread and a good fit of the abutment and casting. In contrast the implant on the right side has a bone level at the second or third thread and a gap between the abutment and casting

• Wide saucerised areas of marginal bone loss visible on radiographs.

This problem will be dealt with in the section on the treatment of peri-implantitis.

Routine hygiene treatment requirements

The patient's oral hygiene should be reviewed and reinforced where necessary. An individual with a healthy dentition and a single tooth implant replacement should have the simplest maintenance requirements and few, if any, complications. The patient should be able to maintain the peri-implant soft and hard tissues in a state of health equivalent to that which exists around their natural teeth, almost without professional intervention (fig. 6). This can be achieved with routine toothbrushing and flossing. However, in some circumstances, the contour of the single tooth restoration is not ideal and instead of producing a smooth readily cleansable emergence profile, poor positioning of the implant may have resulted in a degree of ridge lapping (fig. 7). This will require modification of oral hygiene techniques to clean under the overhanging crown morphology, with dental tape or superfloss passed or threaded under the overhang. Single tooth restorations rarely have calculus formation on their highly

In all cases every effort should be made to minimise distortion and produce comparable reproducible images (see Part 5) to allow longitudinal assessment. Most implant systems report some bone loss in the first year following loading, followed by a steady state in subsequent years in the majority of implants. It would seem reasonable to radiograph annually for the first 3 to 5 years, then bi-annually up to 10 years in the absence of clinical signs or symptoms. If progressive bone loss is detected, the clinician has to decide whether this is most likely caused by bacteria induced inflammation or excessive loading (fig. 5). It may be very difficult to differentiate between the two, and in some circumstances the two factors may be combined.

Occlusal factors are more likely to be implicated in situations where there has been:

• A history of parafunction
• A history of breakages of the superstructure or retaining screws (or screw loosening)
• An angular/narrow pattern of bone loss
• Too few implants placed to replace the missing teeth
• Excessive cantilever extensions.

Bacteria induced factors are more likely to be implicated where there is:

• Poor oral hygiene
• Retention of cement in the subgingival area
• Macroscopic gaps between implant components subgingivally
• Marked inflammation, exudation and proliferation of the soft tissue

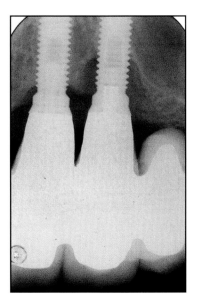

Fig. 5 A periapical radiograph of two implants incorporated in a maxillary bridge. The abutments and casting are well seated. The bone level on the left implant is at the first thread but at the fifth thread on the right implant. The bone loss at the latter implant is quite saucerised. However, it should be noted that the abutment screw in the right implant had previously fractured because of occlusal overload. The apical part of the old screw is visible and the more radiopaque new screw is coronal to this

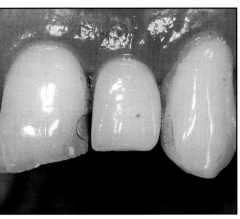

Fig. 6 A single tooth implant replacing an upper lateral incisor. The soft tissue health is very good with no signs of inflammation or bleeding. The patient cares for this unit in the same manner as the natural teeth

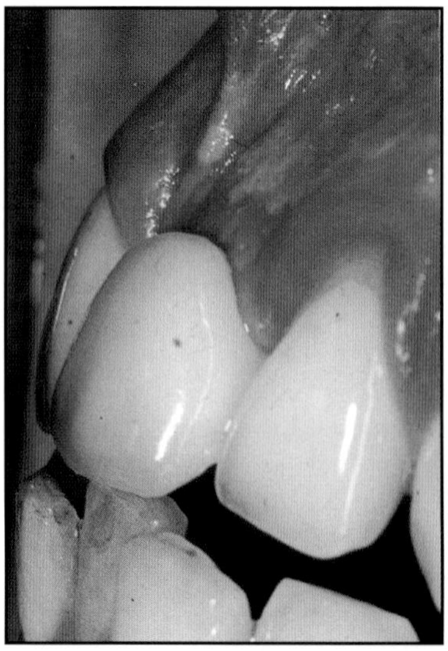

dental implants

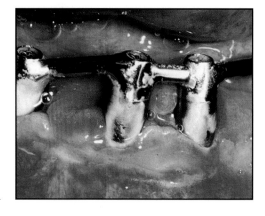

Fig. 7 A single tooth restoration viewed from the side to show a ridge lap profile. This is not ideal and oral hygiene procedures have to be modified to cope with the situation

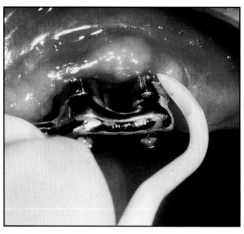

Fig. 8a Calculus will form on titanium abutments

Fig. 8b Plastic scalers rather than stainless steel should be used to remove calculus from titanium surfaces to avoid damage

glazed porcelain or polished gold surfaces. Professional scaling is not therefore normally required.

In patients with more complex fixed or removable prostheses development of readily cleansable embrasure spaces by the technician considerably facilitates patient's oral hygiene. Where calculus deposition has occurred, this should be removed. Calculus should be removed from titanium abutments with instruments which will not damage the surface (fig. 8). In many cases the abutments used are low profile with minimal exposure of the titanium surface subgingivally and this

problem does not arise. Ultrasonic instruments and steel tipped instruments are contra-indicated.

Management of other specific complications

There are a number of complications which require early or urgent treatment.

Implant component failure

Retention and abutment screws which repeatedly loosen suggest either a poor fitting restoration superstructure or excessive loading. These factors require correction and proper management to avoid this complication and this is dealt with in Parts 4 and 7. Failure to deal with these problems, particularly in patients who exhibit parafunctional activities, may predispose to screw fracture (retention screws or abutment screws)(figs 5 and 9).

In many instances the fractured screw can be unwound by engaging the fractured surface with a sharp probe or using a commercially designed retrieval kit. The screw can then be replaced and due attention given to correction of the cause of the problem.

Fortunately, fracture of the implant is rare. It is more likely to occur with:
- Narrow diameter implants, particularly when the wall thickness is thin
- Excessive load
- Marginal bone loss which has progressed to the level of an inherent weakness of the implant, often the level where wall thickness is thin at the apical level of the abutment screw.

Implant fracture is rarely retrievable, and requires either burying the fractured component beneath the mucosa or its removal (fig. 10). The latter can be difficult and traumatic, usually requiring surgical trephining which may leave a considerable defect in the jaw bone.

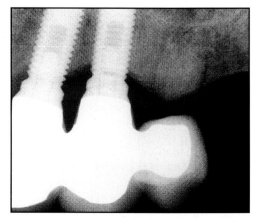

Fig. 9 A periapical radiograph of two implants used to replace three units including a distal cantilever. The abutment screw in the distal implant has fractured. The screw was replaced and the cantilever extension removed

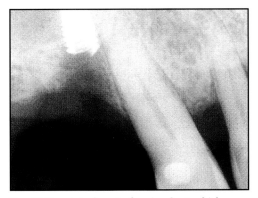

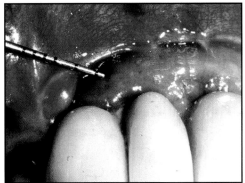

Fig. 11a This patient had repeated soft tissue abscesses and discomfort around the implant supported bridge. The probe shows a soft tissue sinus

Fig. 10 The apical part of an implant which fractured. The implant was short. Overloading and bone loss led to failure

Soft tissue complications

Most inflammatory conditions can be corrected with attention to oral hygiene and professional cleaning. However, there are a number of instances which may require surgical correction:

- Soft tissue overgrowth
- Soft tissue deficiencies
- Persistent inflammation/infection.

Soft tissue proliferation may occur under supporting bars of overdentures. It may require simple excision if there is adequate attached keratinised tissue apical to it, or an inverse bevel resection as used in periodontal surgery to thin out the excess tissue but preserve the keratinised tissue to produce a zone of attached tissue around the abutment. In direct contrast, some patients experience considerable discomfort because of trauma from the removable denture on mobile non-keratinised mucosa surrounding the abutment. The technique of free-gingival grafting can be used to correct this problem (see Part 8). Soft tissue problems may arise because of poor implant positioning. Persistent inflammation or discomfort may require recontouring of the soft tissues to allow patient cleaning, and this may reveal the less than satisfactory aesthetics produced by poor planning and execution of treatment (fig. 11). In other more severe cases the only remedy may be to remove the implants or bury them permanently beneath the mucosa. Poorly designed or constructed prostheses may need to be replaced, but in some cases this would also involve correction of the implant position. A compromise solution may therefore be sought.

Peri-implant lesions

In the case of well documented implants systems, inflammatory peri-implant lesions are rare. The possible aetiology of these lesions was described above and in Part 2. Potential occlusal factors should be diagnosed and corrected. Lesions which are thought to be caused by bacterial colonisation/contamination of the implant surface are managed in a similar fashion to lesions of periodontitis around teeth.

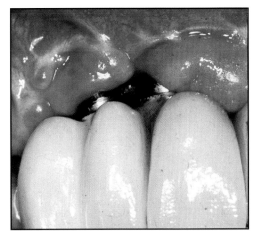

Fig. 11b Soft tissue surgery (as in periodontal surgery) has resulted in apical displacement of the tissue. There is an aesthetic compromise but the patient has better access to clean the under surface of the bridge and around the abutments. The original problem was caused by poor positioning of the implants in the embrasure spaces, rather than under the crowns

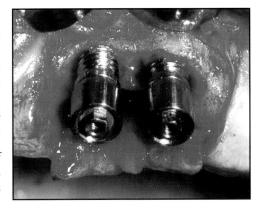

Fig. 12a Elevation of soft tissue from around two implants which had suffered from marginal bone loss and persistent inflammation. The implants surfaces were thoroughly cleaned and the soft tissue sutured at a more apical level (fig. 12b)

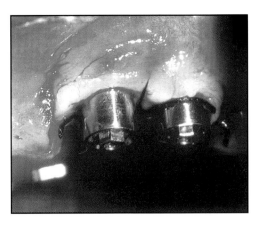

Fig. 12b Flaps sutured at a more apical level to allow improved oral hygiene by the patient

The keratinised mucosa should be preserved as much as possible, by employing an inverse bevel incision to separate it from the underlying inflammatory tissue. Following incision to bone the soft tissue flaps should be elevated to expose normal adjacent bone. The inflammatory tissue surrounding the implant is readily removed (fig. 12). The main difficulty is adequately disinfecting the implant surface. This is more readily accomplished on a relatively smooth surface but may be almost impossible on a very porous surface such as a hydroxyapatite coating. Therefore, rough surfaces require more extensive debridement than a smooth surface which may be adequately disinfected using a topical antiseptic such as chlorhexidine or simple polishing. Inflammatory peri-implant lesions are not sufficiently common to have allowed comparison of different methods of cleaning to promote resolution of the soft tissue inflammation or repair of the bone. In cases where regenerative techniques have been used and bone fill has occurred, there is considerable controversy as to whether or not the regenerated bone forms a new osseointegration with the previously contaminated implant surface.

Conclusions

Regular review and maintenance of patients are essential to maintain the health of implant supporting tissues, to prevent minor complications and measure one's own long-term success at providing this treatment. With meticulous planning, provision of treatment and use of a tried and tested system, the complication rate is low. However, it is important to realise that complications do occur and for patients to appreciate the value of long-term care.

Recommended reading

Adell R, Eriksson B, Lekholm U, Branemark PI & Jemt T (1990). A long-term follow-up study of osseointegrated implants in the treatment of totally edentulous jaws. *International Journal of Oral and Maxillofacial Implants* 5:347-359

Adell R, Lekholm U, Rockler B & Branemark P-I (1981). A 15 year study of osseointegrated implants in the treatment of the edentulous jaw. *International Journal of Oral Surgery* 10:387-416.

Albrektsson T & Sennerby L (1991). State of the art in oral implants. *Journal of Clinical Periodontology* 18: 474-481.

Ali A, Patton DWP, El Sharkawi AMM, Davies J (1997). Implant rehabilitation of irradiated jaws — a preliminary report. *International Journal of Oral and Maxillofacial Implants* 12:523-526.

Andersson B, Odman P & Carlsson GE (1995). A study of 184 consecutive patients referred for single tooth replacement. *Clinical Oral Implants Research* 6:232-237.

Andersson B, Odman P, Lindvall A-M & Branemark P-I (1998). Cemented single crowns on osseointegrated implants after 5 years: Results from a prospective study on CeraOne. *International Journal of Prosthodontics* 11:212-218.

Andersson, B, Odman P, Widmark G. & Waas A (1993). Anterior tooth replacement with implants in patients with a narrow alveolar ridge form. A clinical study using guided tissue regeneration. *Clinical Oral Implants Research* 4:90-98.

Arvidson K, Bystedt H, Frykholm A, von Konow L & Lothigius E (1992). A 3-year clinical study of Astra dental implants in the treatment of edentulous mandibles. *International Journal of Oral and Maxillofacial Implants* 7:321-329.

Arvidson K, Bystedt H, Frykholm A, von Konow L & Lothigius E (1998). Five year prospective follow up report of the Astra Tech implant system in the treatment of edentulous mandibles. *Clinical Oral Implants Research* 9:225-234.

Astrand P (1993). Current implant systems. *Journal of the Swedish Dental Association.* 85:651-663.

Bain CA. (1996). Smoking and implant failure — Benefit of a smoking cessation protocol. *International Journal of Oral and Maxillofacial Implants* 11: 756-759.

Bain CA & Moy PK (1993). The association between the failure of dental implants and cigarette smoking. *International Journal of Oral and Maxillofacial Implants* 8:609-615.

Balshi TJ, Hernandez RE, Pryszlak MC & Rangert B (1996). A comparative study of one implant versus two replacing a single molar. *International Journal of Oral and Maxillofacial Implants.* 11:372-378.

Bahat O & Handelsman M (1996). Use of wide implants and double implants in the posterior jaw: a clinical report. *International Journal of Oral and Maxillofacial Implants.* 11:379-386.

Becker W. & Becker B (1990). Guided tissue regeneration for implants placed into extraction sockets and for implant dehiscences: surgical techniques and case reports. *International Journal of Periodontics and Restorative Dentistry* 10:377-391.

Becker W & Becker BE (1995). Replacement of maxillary and mandibular molars with single endosseous implant restorations. *Journal of Prosthetic Dentistry* 74:51-55.

Bloomqvist JE, Alberius P & Isaksson S (1996). Retrospective analysis of one stage maxillary sinus augmentation with endosseous implants. International *Journal of Oral and Maxillofacial Implants* 11:512-521.

Bragger U (1998). Use of radiographs in evaluating success, stability and failure in implant dentistry. *Periodontology 2000* 4:77-88.

Branemark P-I, Zarb GA & Albrektsson T. eds. (1985) *Osseointegration in clinical dentistry*. Chicago, Quintessence Publishing.

Brown D (1997). All you wanted to know about titanium, but were afraid to ask. *British Dental Journal.* 182:393-394.

ten Bruggenkate CM, Krekeler G, Kraaijenhagen HA, Foitzik C & Osterbeek HS (1993). Haemorrhage of the floor of the mouth resulting from lingual perforation during implant placement: A clinical report. *International Journal of Oral and Maxillofacial Implants* 8: 329-334.

Buser D, Weber HP, Bragger U & Balsiger C (1991). Tissue integration of one-stage ITI implants: 3-year results of a longitudinal study with hollow cylinder and hollow screw implants. *International Journal of Oral and Maxillofacial Implants* 6: 405-412.

Cawood JI & Howell RA (1988). A classification of the edentulous jaws. *International Journal of Oral Maxillofacial Surgery* 1:232-236.

Dahlin C, Andersson L & Linde A (1991). Bone augmentation at fenestrated implants by an osteopromotive membrane technique. A controlled clinical study. *Clinical Oral Implants Research* 2:159-169.

Davis D & Packer M (1999). Mandibular overdentures stabilised by Astra Tech implants with either ball attachments or magnets. *International Journal of Prosthodontics* 12:222-229.

De Bruyn H & Collaert B (1994). The effect of smoking on early implant failure. *Clinical Oral Implants Research* 5:260-264.

Dharmar S (1997). Locating the mandibular canal in panoramic radiographs. *International Journal of Oral and Maxillofacial Implants* 12:113-117.

Eckert S & Wollan P (1998). Retrospective review of 170 endosseous implants placed in partially edentulous jaws. *Journal of Prosthetic Dentistry* 79:415-421.

Ekestubbe A (1993). Reliability of spiral tomography with the Scanora technique for dental implant planning. *Clinical Oral Implants Research* 4: 195-202.

Ellegaard B, Baelum V & Karring T (1997). Implant therapy in periodontally compromised patients. *Clinical Oral Implants Research* 8:180-188.

Ellen R (1998). Microbial colonisation of the peri-implant environment and its longterm success of osseointegrated implants. *International Journal of Prosthodontics* 11:443-441.

Engquist B, Nilson H & Astrand P (1995). Single tooth replacement by osseointegrated Branemark implants. *Clinical Oral Implants Research* 6: 238-245.

Ericsson I, Johansson CB, Bystedt H & Norton MR (1994). A histomorphometric evaluation of bone-to-implant contact on machine-prepared and roughened titanium dental implants. *Clinical Oral Implants Research* 5:202-206.

Eriksson RA & Albrektsson T (1984). The effect of heat on bone regeneration: An experimental study in the rabbit using the bone growth chamber. *Journal of Oral and Maxillofacial Surgery* **42**: 705-711.

Eriksson RA & Adell R (1986). Temperatures during drilling for the placement of implants using the osseointegration technique. *Journal of Oral and Maxillofacial Surgery* **44**: 4-7.

Esposito M, Hirsch JM, Lekholm U & Thomsen P (1998). Biological factors contributing to failures of osseointegrated oral implants: (I) Success criteria and epidemiology. *European Journal of Oral Sciences* **106**:527-551.

Esposito M, Hirsch JM, Lekholm U & Thomsen P (1998). Biological factors contributing to failures of osseointegrated oral implants: (II) Etiopathogenesis. *European Journal of Oral Sciences* **106**:721-764.

Esposito M, Hirsch JM, Lekholm U & Thomsen P (1999). Differential diagnosis and treatment strategies for biologic complications and failing oral implants. *International Journal of Oral and Maxillofacial Implants* **14**:473-490.

Gomez-Roman G, Schulte W, d'Hoedt B & Axman-Krcmar D (1997). The Frialit-2 implant system: five-year clinical experience in single tooth and immediately postextraction applications. *International Journal of Oral and Maxillofacial Implants* **12**: 299-309.

Gotfredsen K, Nimb L, Hjorting-Hansen E, Jensen JS & Holmen A (1992). Histomorphometric and removal torque analysis for TiO2-blasted titanium implants. *Clinical Oral Implants Research* **3**:77-84.

Gunne J, Jemt T, Linden B (1994). Implant treatment in partially edentulous patients: a report on prostheses after 3 years. *International Journal of Prosthodontics* **7**:143-148.

Grondahl K & Lekholm U (1997). The predictive value of radiographic diagnosis of implant instability. *International Journal of Oral and Maxillofacial Implants* **12**: 59-64.

Hammerle CH, Fourmosis I, Winkler JR, Weigel C, Bragger U. & Lang NP (1995). Successful bone fill in late peri-implant defects using guided tissue regeneration. A short communication. *Journal of Periodontology* **66**:303-308.

Hebel K & Gajjar R (1997). Cement retained versus screw retained implant restorations: achieving optimal occlusion and aesthetics in implant dentistry. *Journal of Prosthetic Dentistry* **77**:28-35.

Hobkirk J, Watson RM & Albrektsson T (1995). *Patient assessment in: Dentomaxillofacial Implantology*, London, Mosby Wolfe.

Humphris GM, Healey T, Howell RA & Cawood J (1995). The psychological impact of implant-retained prostheses: a cross-sectional study. *International Journal of Oral and Maxillofacial Implants* **10**:437-444.

Isidor F (1996). Loss of osseointegration caused by occlusal overload of oral implants. *Clinical Oral Implants Research* **7**:143-152.

Isidor F (1997). Histological evaluation of peri-implant bone at implants subjected to occlusal overload or plaque accumulation. *Clinical Oral Implants Research* **8**:1-9.

Ivanoff C-J, Sennerby L & Lekholm U (1996). Influence of initial implant mobility on the integration of titanium implants: An experimental study in rabbits. *Clinical Oral Implants Research* **7**: 120-127.

Jaffin R & Berman C (1991). The excessive loss of Branemark fixtures in type IV bone. *Journal of Periodontology* **62**:2-4.

Jemt T (1998). Customized titanium single-implant abutments: 2 year follow-up pilot study. *International Journal of Prosthodontics* **11**: 312-316.

Jemt T (1994). Fixed implant supported prostheses in the edentulous maxilla. *Clinical Oral Implants Research* **5**:142-147.

Jemt T, Chai J, Harnett J, Heath MR, Hutton JE, Johns RB, McKenna S, McNamara DC, van Steenberghe D, Taylor R, Watson RM & Herrmann I (1996). A 5-year prospective multicenter follow-up report on overdentures supported by osseointegrated implants. *International Journal of Oral and Maxillofacial Implants* **11**:291-298.

Jemt T, Laney W, Harris D, Henry PJ, Krogh PHJ, Polizzi G, Zarb GA & Herrmann I (1991). Osseointegrated implants for single tooth replacement: A 1-year report from a multicenter prospective study. *International Journal of Oral Maxillofacial Implants* **6**:29-36.

Jemt T & Lekholm U (1995) Implant treatment in the edentulous maxilla: a 5 year follow up report on patients with different degrees of jaw resorption. *International Journal of Oral Maxillofacial Implants* **10**:303-311.

Johansson CB & Albrektsson T (1991). A removal torque and histomorphometric study of commercially pure niobium and titanium implants in rabbit bone. *Clinical Oral Implants Research* **2**:24-29.

Kahnberg K-E, Nilsson P & Rasmusson L (1999). Le Fort I osteotomy with interpositional bone grafts and implants for the rehabilitation of the severely resorbed maxilla: a 2-stage approach. *International Journal of Oral and Maxillofacial Implants* **14**:571-578.

Kent G & Johns R (1994). Effects of osseointegrated implants on psychological and social well-being: a comparison with replacement removable prostheses. *International Journal of Oral and Maxillofacial Implants* **9**:103-106.

Laney W, Jemt T, Harris D, Henry PJ, Krogh PHJ, Polizzi G, Zarb GA & Herrmann I (1994). Osseointegrated implants for single tooth replacement: Progress report from a multicenter prospective study after 3 years. *International Journal of Oral Maxillofacial Implants* **6**:29-36.

Lang NP, Karring T & Lindhe J eds (1999) *Proceedings of the 3rd European Workshop on Periodontology: Implant Dentistry*. Quintessence Publishing Co. Berlin.

Langer B, Langer L, Herrmann I & Jorneus L (1993). The wide fixture: a solution for special bone situations and a rescue for the compromised implant. *International Journal of Oral and Maxillofacial Implants* **8**: 400-408.

Lekholm U (1998) Surgical considerations and possible shortcomings of the host sites. *Journal of Prosthetic Dentistry* **79**:43-48.

Lekholm U, Sennerby L, Roos J & Becker W (1996). Soft tissue and marginal bone conditions at osseointegrated implants that have exposed threads: a 5 year retrospective study. *International Journal of Oral and Maxillofacial Implants* **11**:599-604.

Levine RA, Clem DS, Wilson TG, Higginbottom F & Saunders SL (1997). A multicenter retrospective analysis of the ITI implant system used for single-tooth replacements: preliminary results at 6 or more months of loading. *International Journal of Oral and Maxillofacial Implants* **12**:237-242.

Lindh T, Gunne J, Tillberg A & Molin M (1998) A meta analysis of implants in partial edentulism. *Clinical Oral Implants Research* **9**:80-90.

Lindhe J, Karring T & Lang NP eds. (1997) *Clinical Periodontology and Implant Dentistry*. Munksgaard International Publishers. Copenhagen.

Lindquist LW, Carlsson GE & Jemt T (1996) A prospective 15 year follow up study of mandibular fixed prostheses supported by osseointegrated implants. *Clinical Oral Implants Research* **7**:329-336.

Listgarten MA, Lang NP, Shroeder HE & Schroeder A (1991). Periodontal tissues and their counterparts around endosseous implants. *Clinical Oral Implants Research* 2:1-19.

Lundgren S, Moy P, Johansson C & Nilsson H (1996). Augmentation of the maxillary sinus floor with particulate mandible: a histomorphometric study. *International Journal of Oral and Maxillofacial Implants* 11:760-766.

Makkonen TA, Holmberg S, Niemi L, Olsson C, Tammisalo T, & Peltola JA (1997). A 5-year prospective clinical study of Astra Tech dental implants supporting fixed bridges or overdentures in the edentulous mandible. *Clinical Oral Implants Research*, 8: 469-475.

Meredith N (1998). Assessment of implant stability as a prognostic determinant. *International Journal of Prosthodontics* 11:491-501.

Mericske-Stern R, Steinlin Schaffner T, Marti P & Geering AH (1994). Peri-implant mucosal aspects of ITI implants supporting overdentures. A five-year longitudinal study. *Clinical Oral Implants Research* 5:9-18.

Mericske-Stern R, Zarb GA (1993). Overdentures: an alternative implant methodology for edentulous patients. *International Journal of Prosthodontics* 6:203-208.

Millar BJ & Taylor NG (1995). Lateral thinking: the management of missing upper lateral incisors. *British Dental Journal* 179:99-106.

Mombelli A & Lang NP (1992) Antimicrobial treatment of peri-implant infections. *Clinical Oral Implants Research* 3:162-168.

Naert I, Gizani S, Vuylsteke M & van Steenberge D (1998). A 5-year randomized clinical trial on the influence of splinted and unsplinted oral implants in mandibular overdenture therapy. *Clinical Oral Implants Research* 9:17-177.

Norton M (1998) Marginal bone levels at single tooth implants with conical fixture design. The influence of surface macro- and microstructure. *Clinical Oral Implants Research* 9:91-99.

Nyman E, Kahnberg K-E & Gunne J (1993). Bone Grafts and Branemark implants in the treatment of the severely resorbed maxilla: A 2 year longitudinal study. *International Journal of Oral and Maxillofacial Implants* 8:45-53.

Olsson M, Gunne J, Astrand P & Borg K(1995) Bridges supported by free standing implants versus bridges supported by tooth and implant: A five year prospective study. *Clinical Oral Implants Research* 6:114-121.

Oikarinen K, Raustia AM & Hartikainen M (1995). General and local contraindications for endosseal implants — an epidemiological panoramic radiograph study in 65 year old subjects. *Community Dentistry and Oral Epidemiology* 23:114-118.

Palmer RM, Smith BJ, Palmer PJ & Floyd PD (1997). A prospective study of Astra single tooth implants. *Clinical Oral Implants Research* 8:173-179.

Palmer RM, Floyd PD, Palmer PJ, Smith BJ, Johansson CB & Albrektsson T (1994). Healing of implant dehiscence defects with and without expanded polytetrafluoroethylene membranes: a controlled clinical and histological study. *Clinical Oral Implants Research* 5:98-104.

Persson LG, Ericsson I, Berglundh T & Lindhe J (1996). Guided bone regeneration in the treatment of periimplantitis. *Clinical Oral Implants Research* 7:366-372.

Rangert BR, Jemt T & Jorneus L (1989). Forces and moments on Branemark implants. *International Journal of Oral and Maxillofacial Implants* 4: 241-247.

Rangert B, Krogh PH, Langer B & Van Roekel N (1995). Bending overload and implant fracture: a retrospective clinical analysis. International *Journal of Oral and Maxillofacial Implants* 10:326-334.

Reddy S, Mayfield-Donahoo T, Vanderven FJJ & Jeffcoat MK (1994). A comparison of the diagnostic advantages of panoramic radiography and computed tomography scanning for placement of root form dental implants. *Clinical Oral Implants Research* 5:229-238.

Rosenquist B. & Grenthe, B. (1996). Immediate placement of implants into extraction sockets: Implant survival. *International Journal of Oral and Maxillofacial Implants* 11:205-209.

Schenk RK & Buser D (1998). Osseointegration: a reality. *Periodontology 2000* 17:22-35.

Schlumberger T, Bowley JF & Maze GI (1998). Intrusion phenomena in combination tooth implant restorations: a review of the literature. *Journal of Prosthetic Dentistry*. 80:190-203.

Schnitman P, Wohrle PS, Rubenstein JE, DaSilva JD & Wang NH (1997). Ten year results for Branemark implants immediately loaded with fixed bridge prostheses at implant placement. *International Journal of Oral and Maxillofacial Implants* 12:495-503.

Schulte W, d'Hoedt B, Axmann D & Gomez G (1992). The first 15 years of the Tuebingen Implant and its further development to the Frialit -2 system. *Zeitschrift fur Zahnarztliche Implantologie* 8:77-96.

Sennerby L, Ericsson LE, Thomsen P, Lekholm U & Astrand P (1991). Structure of the bone-titanium interface in retrieved clinical oral implants. *Clinical Oral Implants Research* 2:103-111.

Sennerby L & Roos J (1998). Surgical determinants of clinical success of osseointegrated implants: a review of the literature. *International Journal of Prosthodontics* 11:408-420.

Sewerin IP, Gotfredsen K & Stoltze K (1997). Accuracy of radiographic diagnosis of peri-implant radiolucencies- An in vitro experiment. *Clinical Oral Implants Research* 8:299-304.

Sigurdsson TJ, Fu E, Takakis DN, Rohrer MD & Wikesjo UME (1997). Bone morphogenetic protein-2 for peri-implant bone regeneration and osseointegration. *Clinical Oral Implants Research* 8:367-374.

Smith RA, Berger R & Dodson TB (1992). Risk factors associated with dental implants in healthy and medically compromised patients. *International Journal of Oral and Maxillofacial Implants* 7:367-372.

Sonik M, Abrahams J & Faiella RA (1994). A comparison of the accuracy of periapical, panoramic and computerised tomographic radiographs in locating the mandibular canal. *International Journal of Oral and Maxillofacial Implants* 9:455-460.

Steinemann SG (1998). Titanium-the material of choice? *Periodontology 2000* 17:22-35.

Tidwell JK, Blijdorp PA, Stoelinga PJW, Brouns JB & Hinderks F (1992). Composite grafting of the maxillary sinus for placement of endosteal implants – a preliminary report of 48 patients. *International Journal of Oral Maxillofacial Surgery*. 21:204-209.

Tong DC, Rioux K, Drangsholt M & Beirne OR (1998). A review of survival rates for implants in grafted maxillary sinuses using meta-analysis. *International Journal of Oral and Maxillofacial Implants* 13:175-182.

van Steenberghe D, Klinge B, Linden U, Quirynen M, Herrmann I & Garpland C (1993). Periodontal indices around natural and titanium abutments: a longitudinal multicentre study. *Journal of Periodontology* 64:538-541.

van Steenberghe D (1989). A retrospective multicenter evaluation of the survival rate of osseointegrated fixtures supporting fixed partial prostheses in the treatment of partial edentulism. *Journal of Prosthetic Dentistry* 61:217-223.

Von Wowern N (1977). Variations in structure within the trabecular bone of the mandible. *Scandinavian Journal of Dental Research* **85**:478-485.

Von Wowern N (1977). Variations in the bone mass within the cortices of the mandible. *Scandinavian Journal of Dental Research* **85**:444-445.

Watson R & Davis D (1996). Follow up and maintenance of implant supported prostheses: a comparison of 20 complete mandibular dentures and 20 complete fixed cantilever prostheses. *British Dental Journal* **181**:321-327.

Weber HP, Buser D, Donath K, Fiorellini JP, Doppalapudi V, Paquette DW & Williams RC (1996). Comparison of healed tissues adjacent to submerged and non-submerged unloaded titanium dental implants. *Clinical Oral Implants Research* **7**:11-19.

Wennerberg A, Albrektsson T & Andersson B (1993). Design and surface characteristics of 13 commercially available oral implant systems. *International Journal of Oral and Maxillofacial Implants* **8**:622-633

Wennstrom J, Bengazi F & Lekholm U (1994). The influence of the masticatory mucosa on the peri-implant soft tissue condition. *Clinical Oral Implants Research* **5**:1-8.

Westwood RM & Duncan JM (1996). Implants in Adolescents: A review and case reports *International Journal of Oral and Maxillofacial Implants* **11**:750-755.

Wise M (1995) *Failure in the restored dentition: management and treatment.* Quintessence Publishing Co.

Index